25.99

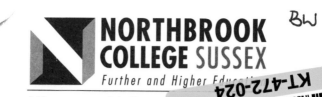

BW

KT-472-024

Partnerships in Health Care

Edited by

Kimmy Eldridge

and

Peter J. Martin

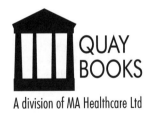

A division of MA Healthcare Ltd

Quay Books Division, MA Healthcare Ltd, St Jude's Church, Dulwich Road, London SE24 0PB

British Library Cataloguing-in-Publication Data
A catalogue record is available for this book

© MA Healthcare Limited 2006

ISBN-10: 1 85642 306 9
ISBN-13: 978 1 85642 306 9

Printed by Athenæum Press Ltd, Dukesway, Team Valley, Gateshead, Tyne & Wear NE11 0PZ

Contents

Foreword

Professor Christine Beasley, Chief Nursing Officer

I was delighted to be invited to provide a foreword for this book because partnerships are such an important aspect of my work as Chief Nursing Officer. The establishment and maintenance of partnerships is a cornerstone of policy, not just in health, but also in all government departments. This book adds to this current policy direction and debates how we can continually improve partnerships at all levels of provider organisations. The importance of partnerships within health care should not be understated, and I am pleased that those who have contributed to this book are exploring best practice. The NHS is a dynamic organisation and the issues raised in the following pages offer many and varied points to be considered as we deliver health care in the next decades.

Good quality nursing, midwifery and health visiting are integral to health care in the UK; and professional development is an important component of delivering this provision. I applaud the efforts of the nurses who have contributed to this book. They have all endeavoured to carry out original work that challenges and expands our understanding of partnerships. This work shows a strong commitment to personal and professional development and these nurses are an example to all health care workers.

The book also demonstrates in itself a form of partnership, between Higher Education Institutions (HEIs) and NHS Trusts. A good quality partnership between these institutions ensures that Trusts have access to the knowledge, skills and resources of HEIs and that HEIs understand the current issues and concerns facing health care providers in the 21st century. This book, as the product of a partnership between the editors at the University of Essex and the authors based in local NHS trusts, demonstrates just what can be achieved by working together.

I hope you will be inspired, motivated and challenged by what you read in this book. You may find that you are inspired to examine how partnerships work in your own organisation. You may also find that you are motivated to examine how partnerships may be improved and how patients and service users might become involved in this process. If you are challenged by what you read then you are engaging with this important debate about how health and social care are delivered now and in the future.

Preface

The papers collected together in this book have been assembled with the intention of demonstrating the importance of partnership in contemporary health care settings. The book examines the principles and practice of partnerships as they are realised by practitioners. In so doing it explores the use of the term 'partnership' as a guiding principle and critically examines its merit. Partnership is not a single and unified concept for which there is common understanding. It is a term that has entered the language and is applied liberally within a range of contexts to express a variety of endeavours. The book explores how the different writers define and apply the term and establishes whether comparable principles are recognisable in each case.

The contributors to the book were all students on an MSc scheme of the University of Essex. They have all since qualified and some have gone on to further academic study. The work that this group of students produced for this scheme was assessed as being of a very high standard by internal and external examination, and it was proposed that the work should be brought to the attention of the wider health care community. The editors identified work around the theme of partnership and invited students to present their work in a suitable form for publication.

The structure of the book grew out of discussion between the researchers and the editors. The editors were responsible for providing the structure, which consists of chapters containing papers that share a common focus: Users and Providers, Mental Health, Information Giving, and Service Partnerships. The editors examine the papers to trace common partnership themes, which are used to construct the concluding chapter. The conclusion examines the implications for partnership working in contemporary practice and shows how partnership is currently understood and practised by health care professionals.

Editing the work of nine authors has necessitated a degree of compromise and order. Each paper is approximately one quarter of its original length; the editors, working with the authors, have attempted to maintain the coherency of each paper. Inevitably, however, some of the detail has been lost. The papers are presented in a systematic manner to aid readability. It should be noted that the original papers might not have used the heading and structure imposed upon the papers during the editing process.

We hope that you will find the contents of this book useful and the structure accessible. The term 'partnership' is widely used throughout the health and social services. It is applied to different contexts and with different intentions. This book contributes to the debate by expanding our understanding of the term as it is used in contemporary practice settings. It also provides evidence of the enactment of policy through changing practices. The book provides detailed exemplars of 'real' partnerships in health and social care, which readers can explore further with a view to developing their own practice and the practice of others.

Kimmy Eldridge and Peter J. Martin
June 2006

Contributors

Elizabeth Carpenter
Liz is a currently a Consultant Nurse in Critical Care. She has extensive experience working within the field of critical care, within both intensive and acute care. This has involved her working collaboratively across professional and organisational boundaries and within Higher Education to support and develop acute and critical care practice. She obtained an MSc in Advanced Clinical Practice in 2004 and she is currently undertaking a Doctorate in Nursing at the University of Essex.

Susan Eastbrook
Susan qualified as an RGN in 1975 at St Bartholomew's Hospital. She has worked within acute general nursing as a night sister and ward manager before commencing the role of patient care coordinator for medicine. Sue, along with her colleague Debbie Reynolds, was asked to pilot and develop her current role, the first of its kind to be introduced in the UK. The role has improved patient pathways of care during emergency admission. It has also improved the interface between, medicine, nursing and diagnostic departments.

Kimmy Eldridge
Professor Kimmy Eldridge was born in Malaysia and has lived and worked in the UK since 1967. She is responsible, at the University of Essex, for strategic development, interpreting professional and government policies, and advising the University and NHS partners on the education and training of health care professionals. In addition the Eastern Deanery employs Kimmy to organise the Colchester General Practitioner (GP) Vocational Training. In this role she takes part in the recruitment and selection of GP trainees and in approval visits to GPs and their practices to determine their suitability to provide placement-based learning.

Moira Keating
Moira is stroke care coordinator at Colchester General Hospital, a role that entails coordinating multi-agency services for stroke care. She qualified as a SRN in 1979 and attained a BA in 1999. In 2002 she was awarded an MSc from the University of Essex. Moira has maintained a professional interest in reha-

bilitation nursing for much of her nursing career and has worked specifically in stroke care for ten years.

Peter J. Martin
Peter is a senior lecturer at the University of Essex. He leads the Professional Doctorate schemes in health and social care in the Department of Health and Human Sciences. As a mental health nurse, he practices within the local mental health Trust working in groups with people who have enduring mental health problems. He is particularly interested in recovery and the subjective experience of mental illness. Peter completed his doctorate in 1999, which examined influences on the clinical judgement of mental health nurses.

Deborah Reynolds
Debbie qualified as RGN in 1983 at Colchester General Hospital. She worked in acute general nursing as a night sister and managed an acute medical ward for older people before taking up the post of patient care coordinator. Debbie, along with her colleague Sue Eastbrook, was asked to pilot and develop her current role, the first of its kind to be introduced in the UK. The role has improved patient pathways of care during emergency admission. It has also improved the interface between medicine, nursing and diagnostic departments.

Diane Treadwell
Diane currently works as a Nurse Practitioner in a busy South Essex practice. She trained and worked at The Royal London Hospital between 1987 and 1997 where she developed a passion for medicine. Diane became interested in the way Primary Care worked and moved into Practice Nursing whilst doing her first degree. Diane's main interest now is working with people who live with cardiac and respiratory conditions.

Rachel 'Ray' Wilson
Ray is the Deputy Director of Community and Day Services at St Helena Hospice in Colchester. From 1978 to 1981 Ray studied music at Colchester Institute for Higher Education. A career change meant that she qualified as a nurse at the North East Essex School of Nursing in 1986. Ray has 19 years' experience in cancer nursing. In 2004, she completed an MSc in Advanced Clinical Practice (Palliative Care) at the University of Essex.

Nick Wrycraft
Nick is currently employed as a Senior Lecturer in mental health by Anglia Ruskin University and is a student on the Professional Doctoral programme at the University of Essex. On qualifying as a mental health nurse Nick gained wide experience of adult and elderly mental health services before moving on

to work as a research facilitator in primary care. His interests include clinical supervision, mental health in primary care settings and service design.

Jane Young

Jane is currently employed as the Lead Diabetes Nurse Specialist working with a team of Diabetes Specialist Nurses based at Broomfield Hospital, Chelmsford. Jane has a background in acute medicine in varied clinical settings and has worked abroad in Denmark and Hong Kong. Particular areas of interest are the impact of culture on health care delivery and patient education. Outside of work, Jane is driven by a passion for sailing and exploring remote parts of the world.

Introduction

Rosy Stamp, Director, St Helena Hospice, Colchester

I am delighted to introduce a book about partnership, a theme that is dear to the heart of St Helena Hospice. We are most grateful to the authors of the book, all local health practitioners and academics, for donating the proceeds to this Hospice.

Dame Cicely Saunders first began to attend to the need for a holistic, less medicalised, service for patients with incurable disease in 1967, with the establishment of St Christopher's Hospice in Sydenham. The United Kingdom has continued to lead the way in developing appropriate services for those who require palliative care. Partnership working is integral to such organisations and the hospice movement continually strives to achieve better standards for those who use our services. Hospices focus on listening to patients and working in partnership with families; they are role models in patient-centred working.

Most hospices are independent voluntary organisations that emerge like mushrooms within their local communities. They are truly community organisations – held in high regard and with a sense of pride and ownership from their local community. The community provides not only financial support but also the volunteers who give of their time and skills. Most hospices are small organisations that achieve high standards through the immediacy of their management and governance. The involvement of the community throughout the organisation promotes openness and accountability and has given hospice founders and supporters a strong voice in the growth and development of their own organisation. Patients and family members have also felt empowered in a way that is unusual within an NHS organisation. Hospices have, therefore, been partners with local members of the public and patients to an extent that would be unusual in many organisations.

Small, independent organisations working in isolation, no matter how successful and well regarded, must always be self-evaluating. Vulnerable patients need all those caring for them to be communicating effectively. This is especially so in palliative care, where time is of the essence and a day missed or a message not passed on may mean that a patient is denied care or support at the end of life. In recent years, hospices such as St Helena have tried to reach out into their local health communities and to build relationships, developing services in response to local health needs. The need to work in partnership with the NHS through Primary Care Trusts and Acute Trusts is pragmatic as well as philosophical, especially as we move towards further health care reorganisations and commissioning. We are enthusiastically committed to developing mutually supportive relationships locally and to becoming increasingly responsive to, and collaborative with, others in the local health environment.

For all of us though, our key partnerships must be with patients. We are moving into an era where patient choice is not just good practice, but also government policy. This is an exciting opportunity for all of us working in health care to reflect on our own practice and to learn from our patients how we can move forward into a relationship based on true partnership.

The health care environment has, until recently, been infamous for relationships based on an imbalance of power. In 1660, Samuel Pepys was tied to a table and held down by strong men to have his kidney stone removed; desperate people will put up with desperate measures. Mental health patients have been medicated against their will, parents' and children's rights to have contact with each other have been refused for specious medical reasons, and even bereaved parents' rights to consent over their children's body parts have recently and notoriously been ignored. Doctors throughout the last century were frequently god-like figures, attended by subservient nurses and other staff, with patients viewed as a collection of systems and symptoms rather than sentient beings. It is relatively recently that medical staff have been encouraged to view themselves as team members, working in interdisciplinary teams where each member has an equally valid input. Such a profound revision of self-image takes time and the traditional dominance of medicine still pervades many older hospitals.

As for patients themselves, we talk about patient choice and great efforts are made by some clinical teams to communicate effectively and to look after the psychological and emotional needs of the patient. It is sad that patients, all too often, still feel like an inconvenience, an interruption to the day of a health care worker. Emotional and spiritual needs remain unmet because they are seen as less important than physical health needs. Patients are still flooded with jargon, leaving appointments with questions unanswered and more full of apprehension than when they arrived. Knowledge is power, and too often patients do not have the knowledge that would allow them to be more assertive in their use of health care professionals and systems. It is exciting to see patients becoming empowered through access to good information and through groups where they can support each other. We show our commitment to these principles through our Partnership Group and representation on our Board of Trustees and Clinical Governance Group from users at this Hospice.

So, in conclusion, what does partnership imply? First of all, it indicates equality between people and not a relationship where one person is dominant. Secondly, it implies a cooperative relationship, where people gain from each other and have investment in effective collaboration and communication. To achieve true partnership there need to be harmony of purpose and true mutual respect.

CHAPTER I

An overview of health care partnerships in the United Kingdom

This chapter provides an overview of partnership working in the UK health care setting to provide the context for subsequent chapters. It is not a systematic review, rather a review based on selected literature (including commentaries).

Part I
An overview of partnership in UK general health care
Kimmy Eldridge

Intention

To examine:

- The problematic nature of partnership as a concept
- The drivers and barriers to partnership working in the UK health care setting
- The achievements in partnership working

Definition and purpose

Partnership is a term that is seen as being central to the Government's public services policy. Consistent with its electoral pledges in 1997 to improve the quality of health care, the Labour Government has set out its vision for a new and modern NHS. The competition culture, created by the internal market under the previous government, was to be replaced with partnership (Department of

Health, 1997). This was to be achieved by 'breaking down organisational barriers and forging stronger links with local authorities' (Department of Health, 1997). Openness and public involvement were to become a key feature of all parts of the new NHS; in particular, the Government emphasised that 'the needs of the patient not the needs of institutions will be at the heart of the new NHS' (Department of Health, 1997).

The ten-year NHS Plan (Department of Health, 2000a) made clear that increased funding from the public purse would be tied to service reform and modernisation. The suggestion that these changes were necessary to modernise the NHS and put patients at its centre is highly emotive; by implication, those questioning change are at risk of being seen as working against patients' interests.

While these policy statements proved effective tools to motivate and energise NHS staff, the language used and the speed with which the policies were introduced did not encourage national debate. Managers continue to concentrate on waiting time and other performance targets which, it could be argued, preclude patient-centredness and longer consultation. Moreover, the policy drive towards partnership working in health and social care is not new. Successive governments have attempted to bring health and social services together since the early 1960s, but without success (Hudson and Henwood, 2002).

Conservative as well as Labour governments encouraged purchaser–provider relationships (later commissioner and provider) based on trust and collaboration. However, this policy objective is inconsistent with the requirement of organisations to drive down the cost of health and social care with competitive tendering (Hudson and Henwood, 2002). At an organisational level, one of the barriers to inter-agency collaboration is the absence of a single health and social care budget. The health and social care division thus prevents access to a seamless service designed to meet the needs of the individual.

The 1999 Health Act made partnership a statutory duty of all NHS organisations (Department of Health, 1997) in an effort to break down the 'Berlin Wall' between health and social care. However, the term 'partnership' was not defined (Hudson and Henwood, 2002; McLaughlin, 2004; Tomlinson, 2005). Furthermore, it was used interchangeably with 'collaborative approach' (Department of Health, 1997). This ambiguity allows for local interpretation and implementation and makes systematic evaluation of partnership development difficult.

The literature suggests that there is no universally accepted definition of partnership (McLaughlin, 2004; Wildridge *et al.*, 2004; Tomlinson, 2005). Nonetheless, the literature suggests that partnership includes the following elements (McLaughlin, 2004; Wildridge *et al.*, 2004):

- Shared aims, goals or vision between individuals, groups and organisations
- Joint rights, resources and responsibilities
- Autonomy and interdependence

- New structures and processes
- Trust
- Improved and enhanced access to services for users and carers

One of the main perceived benefits of partnership working is that the partners are able to share ideas, knowledge and resources (McLaughlin, 2004).

Organisational level partnership

Primary Care Trusts (PCTs) are an example of organisational partnership. PCTs bring together all GPs and community nurses within a specific local area to improve the health of the local community by providing integrated primary care services and commissioning secondary care. By 2002, five years after the Labour Government came into office, 303 PCTs were established in England. Eighty per cent of NHS funding was redirected to PCTs on a capitation-based formula, that is, a system of allocating funding based on the needs of the local population (Walsh *et al.*, 2004).

PCTs were legally required to form strong links with social services and to have a governing body with representation from community nursing, social services and GPs. Locally focused activity such as Health Action Zones and Health Improvement Programmes (which are action programmes led by the health authority involving NHS organisations, health care professionals, local authorities and other local agencies) were intended to support partnership working further. There was high expectation that PCTs would deliver a clinically driven and locally responsive service (Department of Health, 1997).

Most commentators who had previously criticised the lack of coordination between health and social care (Rummery, 1999; Clark and Glendinning, 2002) welcomed the measures to foster stronger working relationships. However, despite an unprecedented investment in the second term of the Labour Government to drive change and partnership working in health and social care, there was no dedicated funding to evaluate its implementation. Nonetheless, small-scale research findings show that representation at PCT board level has had a generally positive effect on inter-professional and inter-agency relationships (Coleman and Rummery, 2003).

Many PCTs are sharing expertise and functions with neighbouring organisations. However, health and social services planning and commissioning remain fragmented (Coleman and Rummery, 2003). As immature organisations, PCTs require further time to develop their commissioning capability. PCTs are currently perceived by policy makers and critics as ineffective organisations that have failed to develop credible management teams that can stand up to the well-established hospital trusts when negotiating and commissioning services (Gould, 2004). PCTs are also criticised for being too small to fulfil their public health responsibilities (Walsh *et al.*, 2004). In effect, PCTs fall far short of the Government's ambitions and partnership largely remains a paper-filling exercise (Rummery, 2003).

Halfway through the ten-year NHS Plan, the Government announced yet another structural change (Department of Health, 2005a). Strategic health authorities and ambulance trusts are to merge, and the number of PCTs will be reduced and their function altered. The changes began in 2006. Improving patient care, empowering front-line staff and saving unnecessary management costs are the planned benefits. In reality, as research into managing partnership in primary care shows, service delivery and partnership working will be compromised by the pace of change, targets and performance measures (Charlesworth, 2001). The new organisations and staff need time to develop the interpersonal trust that is essential for effective partnership (Lowndes *et al.*, 1997; Tomlinson, 2005).

Mergers, another form of partnership, have been known to set back organisations in terms of services development by at least 18 months (Garside, 1999; Fulop *et al.*, 2002). International studies have found no conclusive evidence of the benefits of mergers and the influence of hospital size on the quality, cost of, and access to health care (NHS Centre for Review and Dissemination, 1997). Observers conclude that policy makers in the UK may be using service reconfigurations to reduce bed numbers and discipline stubborn clinicians and weak managers who fail to control costs (Sheldon and Maynard, 1999).

The Nuffield Institute for Health has developed a Partnership Assessment Tool to measure the success of partnership working. The six principles underpinning the Tool are (Hardy *et al.*, 2000):

1. Realism of the purpose of the partnership
2. Acknowledgement of the need for partnership
3. Commitment and ownership
4. Development and maintenance of trust
5. Clear and robust partnership arrangements
6. Monitoring, review and organisational learning

Partnership in the NHS, when it is centrally driven, often fails to fulfil the above criteria at the beginning of the partnership (Tailby *et al.*, 2004). Research has found that initially primary care organisations were more concerned with developing internal structures and commissioning than with acknowledging the need for partnership working with local social services. However, as these organisations matured, their focus changed and partnership working became more of a mainstream activity. Trusting relationships between professionals need time to develop (Rummery, 2003).

Clinical partnerships, such as the Cancer Collaborative Services Project, are another initiative of the Department of Health (Kelly, 2001). These partnerships were established to pool expertise and share expensive equipment in specific areas of care, and require clinicians to work across organisational boundaries. Initially, most clinicians were lured by the prospect of substantial increases in service funding, but most have now become strong supporters of this way of working (Kelly, 2001).

Partnership at professional level

The government policy of placing the patient at the centre of care requires health care staff to abandon traditional boundaries and power struggles in order to focus on patient needs (Department of Health, 2000a). This is problematic, as poor team communication and working is one of the most commonly identified causes of a reduced ability to deliver quality care (Health Service Ombudsman for England, 1998, 2001, 2002).

The extent to which team working is a problem is best illustrated by the way in which information about patients is collected and recorded. In 1995, the Audit Commission identified that as many as 25 professionals may contribute to the care of one patient admitted to hospital with a myocardial infarction (Audit Commission, 1995). Thus the patient is potentially subjected to being questioned 25 times as each profession collects and records information in medical records, nursing records, physiotherapy records and so on.

It has been found that clinical documentation can take up to 25% of a nurse's time in an acute care setting (Smeltzer *et al.*, 1996). Cumulatively, in the year 1995/6, the amount of time that UK doctors spent documenting information they had collected on admissions, day cases and new outpatient attendances was estimated as being equal to approximately 2500 medical whole time equivalents (Clinical Systems Group, 1998). However, efforts to introduce an integrated, single patient record failed because doctors rejected nursing entries as irrelevant and a hindrance to accessing vital information in an emergency (Eldridge and Ramkhelawon, 1999). In addition, physiotherapy and occupational therapy have maintained that it is absolutely critical to their practice that they hold their profession-specific patient records in their department (Eldridge and Ramkhelawon, 1999).

The Bristol Enquiry (Kennedy, 2001) into the care of children receiving complex surgical services found that the staff cared greatly about human suffering and were dedicated and well motivated. However, despite their good intentions, they failed to communicate with each other and to work together effectively in the interests of their patients. The following abstract from the report describes the nature of the problem (Kennedy, 2001):

At the time, consultants, particularly the surgeons, saw themselves as having very effective teams. But they saw these as their team, which they led. They are not part of the team, other than leaders. Also, the teams were teams of 'like professionals', consultant surgeons leading surgeons, consultant anaesthetists leading anaesthetists. The team were not organised primarily around the care of the patient. They were not cross speciality or multi-disciplinary, and they were profoundly hierarchical.

The inability of the doctors in Bristol to work across both speciality and multi-disciplinary boundaries is not unique (National Confidential Enquiry into Peri-operative Deaths, 2002). However, a health service that focuses on the needs of the patient demands a particular type of team working. The literature suggests that holistic patient-centred care will only be achieved where there is true inter-professional working with a sharing of responsibility and pooling of resources, and where team members recognise the core expertise of each other (Laidler, 1994; Ovretveit *et al.*, 1997).

It has been found that it is particularly difficult for doctors to recognise and respect the expertise of other professions. Jorm and Kam (2004) state that the process of training medical specialists develops doctors as reluctant team players, fearing that team work will lead to loss of autonomy, power, status and potential income. Doctors' legal responsibility for patients will continue to be a significant factor in the power relations between the doctor and other health care professions, including nurses (Sweet and Norman, 1995).

The dominance of doctors over nurses, and the subtle and covert way in which nurses influence medical decisions, was first described by Stein in 1967 as 'the doctor–nurse game'. Stein and his colleagues revisited this subject in 1990 and found that the decreasing public regard for doctors, the increasing number of female doctors and male nurses and the recognition by the medical profession of its fallibility have all helped to change the nature of the doctor–nurse relationship; nurses are being valued and regarded with increased esteem in their own right rather than as doctors' assistants. Moreover, the movement of nurse training from hospital to university has helped to shift the power dynamic between doctors and nurses (Mackay, 1993).

Inter-professional learning is now an important quality indicator of health professional education in the UK. Education commissioners and the Department of Health are encouraging education providers to create opportunities for shared learning where recruits to health care disciplines learn to work as a team and develop team-working skills. The Department of Health has a dedicated website to promote this aspect of professional education (Department of Health, 2006a).

At one level, expanded nursing roles are a testimony to improved relationships and collaboration between doctors and nurses. Among some of the recently developed roles is that of the Critical Care Practitioner (CCP) at Papworth Hospital, Cambridge, which was developed jointly by a senior surgical registrar and senior nursing staff of the intensive care unit. The CCPs make all decisions about routine clinical management for 80% of patients who have an uncomplicated recovery following routine cardiac surgery (English, 1997).

Another comparable development was at the Great Ormond Street Hospital for Children in London. Nurses were trained to take over the combined roles of anaesthetist, perfusionist and intensivist while providing conventional nursing care. The consultant intensivist now prefers to work directly with these specialist nurses, rather than with inexperienced junior doctors in rotation (English, 1997).

Such roles span the practice domains of medicine and nursing, challenging role boundaries and traditions and, as such, demand trust. They necessitate the contribution of both professions in the planning and management of the role's development (Dowling *et al.*, 1996). The examples cited here reflect the attributes of inter-professional working as identified by Laidler (1994) and Ovretveit *et al.* (1997); professionals who embrace inter-professional working are confident enough in their own role and professional identity to share and defer their professional autonomy in order to work together.

Notwithstanding the contribution of such new roles, there are concerns among nurses that such developments, which are mainly technical and task-oriented, compromise the essence of nursing and caring (English, 1997; Radcliffe, 2000). Moreover, critics see such developments as just a means to enable the implementation of EU working time directives (English, 1997), pulling nurses away from relating to patients in a caring way and not serving the interests of nursing development (Frank, 2002). Such criticism is based on the observation that certain partnership developments are not driven by doctors and nurses themselves as a way of meeting local needs, but are rather driven by financial and other resource pressures. The rationale is that it makes policy and management sense to transfer work from doctors, who are paid more, to nurses, who are paid less (Richardson and Maynard, 1995).

It is feared that these new roles, which involve medical supervision, may reinforce the traditional handmaiden role of the nurse (Denner, 1995; Williams *et al.*, 1997). However, some nurses argue that working closely with their colleagues enables the development of a collegiate relationship, and allows them to disagree openly with medical decisions (Price and Williams, 2003).

The nurse consultant role, which spans both medical and nursing boundaries, was created by the Department of Health in order to provide a clinical career ladder for nurses (Department of Health, 1999a). There is, as yet, no research evidence on the impact of the role on patient care. Descriptive research reveals that nurse consultants who lack experience in clinical, teaching and research practice and are not educated to at least a master's degree standard are more likely to feel inferior or unequal to doctors (Woodward *et al.*, 2005).

Since the 1990s, and the introduction of the general practitioner (GP) contracts that included payment for health promotion and chronic disease management, GPs have delegated health promotion and disease management work to nurses (Charles-Jones *et al.*, 2003). More recently, a small but increasing number of nurse practitioners are becoming partners in general practice. These nurse partners have the same status and rights as a GP partner. GPs have acknowledged the advantages of this arrangement; as one GP has stated:

> Being a partner means that she [the nurse] is at the heart of decision making within the practice. In addition, she has the financial incentive of being a partner because she will be buying into the property and will be taking in profit share.... She is like an extra GP in the practice but, being a nurse, she comes at things from a slightly different angle.

The GPs reported that having extra support has enabled them to extend their average appointment time from 7 to 15 minutes. The Nursing Doctorate completed by the nurse has also benefited the practice as a whole; they now have enhanced organisational and team building skills (Benson, 2005).

The fact that GPs, as businessmen, are prepared to have nurses as business partners and to share their profit is undoubtedly a giant step towards GPs recognising the contribution of a nursing perspective in partners' meetings and organisational decision making. This arrangement will also benefit patient care.

Partnership with patients

The Government's demands that the NHS must become patient-centred have provoked a degree of consternation among, most particularly, doctors, who feel that such an assertion denies their already existent dedication and commitment to patient care (Smith, 2003). However, the medical press has recognised that a doctor–patient partnership means more than dedication and caring, it is about working with patients in collaboration (MacGregor, 1998; Mariotto, 1999).

Charles *et al.* (1999) proposed three theoretical treatment decision-making models:

- The **paternalistic**: based on the assumption that doctors, drawing on medical knowledge, will be able to act in the best interest of patients without involving them in the decision-making process.
- The **informed**: a model in which the key role and responsibility of the doctor is to provide sufficient information for the patient to make decision. The

premise of this model is that the patient's reference in treatment decision matters more than that of the doctor's.

▦ The **shared**: both the doctor and the patient have a legitimate investment in the treatment decision. The role of the doctor is to create an environment in which patients feel comfortable to express their treatment preference.

Charles *et al.* (1999) suggest that the form of partnership adopted depends on the specific clinical context as well as patient and doctor preference. In a medical emergency and when the patient is unconscious and there is no relative available, a paternalistic model is undoubtedly appropriate. In high-risk surgery and end-of-life decisions, it is the prerogative of the patient to exercise choice. However, the General Medical Council's (GMC) guidelines permit doctors to withdraw artificial nutrition or hydration from patients if doctors think that the quality of life of the patient is very poor (Dyer, 2005). This paternalistic approach was successfully challenged in July 2004 by Lesley Burke; Mr Justice Munby ruled that it is up to patients, not doctors to decide what was in their best interest (*The Times*, 2004). Some doctors were appalled by such a ruling:

Opening the floodgate to patients demanding all sorts of treatments that theoretically prolong life, but are expensive and possibly downright dangerous, undermining the specialist role of the medical professionals in making expert decisions (Anthony-Pillai, 2004).

The judge doesn't seem to have thought through the implication... in short, this could be the end of evidence-based medicine as we know it (Rumbold, 2004).

Most doctors recognise that moving away from a paternalistic model to shared and informed decision making requires more than just funding. Both doctors and patients will need training if these decision-making models are to be achieved (Richards, 1998; Mariotto, 1999; Kennedy *et al.*, 2005).

In an attempt to forge partnerships with patients, the Government introduced the notion of the 'expert patient' in 1999 (Department of Health, 1999b). The Expert Patient Programme is based on the statistic that one in three people in the UK has a chronic disease or disability and that they are the ones who are most informed about how best to manage their condition (Department of Health, 1999b). The aim of the Expert Patient Programme is to develop patients' confidence and skills to work in partnership with health professionals and to improve quality of life (Department of Health, 1999a).

The use of the term *expert* in the context of the expert patient assumes a definition where knowledge and understanding are derived from experience and not education. However, the term is usually reserved for those who have completed appropriate education and socialisation, a process linked to the application of scientific rules and analysis (Wilson, 2001). The medical profession has been sceptical about the initiative. For many doctors the term *expert patient* conjures up an image of a patient clutching a print-out from the Internet, and demanding treatment for which there is no evidence of effectiveness (Shaw and Baker, 2004). A survey found that 58% of doctors predicted that the expert patient initiative will increase GPs' workloads and 42% believe it will increase NHS costs, while only 12% think that it will improve the doctor–patient relationship (Association of the British Pharmaceutical Industry, 1999). Doctors are still debating the appropriateness of the term *expert patient*. There have been calls to replace it with less intimidating and provocative terms such as 'autonomous', 'resourceful' and 'involved' (Shaw and Baker, 2004).

International research has found that enabling patients to self-manage their condition makes less demands and better use of health professionals' time, with, in some cases, a reduction of up to 42–44% of visits to doctors (Lorig *et al.*, 1999; Barlow *et al.*, 2000). Despite such tentative evidence, critics of the policy warn that having a chronic disease does not inevitably mean that a person wants to be an expert patient. Individuals' readiness is influenced by past life experiences, as well as health care professionals' responses to, and society's expectations of, them (Wilson, 2001).

The notion of the expert patient is at odds with three long-held beliefs about the power relationship between patients and professionals:

* First, that the professional not the patient is the expert.
* Second, that the professional is the legitimate gatekeeper to all health care services.
* Third, that the patient is both compliant and self-reliant (Wilson 2001).

If the expert patient initiative is to succeed, the imbalance of power between health professionals and patients must be redressed and the fact that health professionals are skilled at disempowering patients recognised (Taylor, 2000). The literature is full of such examples: GPs who do not follow the guidelines for removing patients from their lists and who permit only one problem per consultation (saving the rest for future appointments) (Taylor, 2000); and nurses using persuasion to ensure that patients conform to their understanding of appropriate behaviour, labelling those who do not as 'difficult patients' (Hewison, 1995).

Another measure that has been introduced by the Department of Health to foster professional patient partnerships is the introduction of the concept of concordance. It describes the agreement between a patient and a health care professional about whether, when and how medicines should be taken (Marinker and Shaw, 2003). The concept has replaced the notion of compliance in the taking of medicines, which implied coercion on the part of the health care professional and passive obedience on the part of the patient (Heath, 2003; White, 2003). When a prescribed medication is not producing the expected benefits, doctors take the decision to change the dosage or prescribe an alternative medication (Marinker and Shaw, 2003). However, patients have their own beliefs about medicine, and link to these beliefs their attitudes to health and health care, risk and benefits, including taking or stopping medication (Britten, 1994). Health care professionals should therefore accept that a patient's decision not to accept treatment is not negative behaviour (Connect, 2000) or failure to comply, but rather a lack of concordance.

The main criticism of concordance is that it does not take into account the fact that at times compliance may be required to safeguard the health of others, as in the case of tuberculosis and human immunodeficiency virus (HIV) (Heath, 2003). All the criticism associated with concordance highlights the inevitability of divergent views about health. Although concordance promotes patients' views, it also supports the assumption that medical knowledge is more valid and reliable than the lay person's (Wilson, 2001). Medical observers, therefore, suggest that if patients have to accept the primacy of medical knowledge, then concordance is merely 'a wolf in sheep's clothing' and is no different from compliance (Heath, 2003).

Policy influences aside, GPs in the UK have, since the 1960s, aspired to move away from scientific, biomedical and hospital-based medicine to a biographical approach to care (Charles-Jones *et al.*, 2003). Such approaches are inherently patient-centred and value the patient's narrative in the consultation. The postgraduate vocational training for doctors to become GPs and the Royal College of General Practitioners' membership examination assess the extent to which GPs are patient-centred in consultation. The criteria of assessment include the ability of doctors to (Campion *et al.*, 2002):

- Follow the patient's cues
- Explore the patient's own beliefs about the illness
- Check the patient's understanding
- Provide patient choice in the consultation

Nonetheless, research has found that doctors at the end of a three-year postgraduate GP training programme showed limited ability to achieve patient-centred outcomes (Campion *et al.*, 2002). Moreover, general practice frequently fails to meet the aspirations of the biographical medicine ideology (Dowrick *et al.*, 1996; May *et al.*, 1996). Some observers claim that the Government's obsession about throughput and waiting times will prevent GPs from delivering holistic patient care (Charles-Jones *et al.*, 2003). It is argued that the criteria used to determine patients' access to appropriate health care only focus on patients' biomedical needs, and there is no scope for considering their psychosocial circumstances (Charles-Jones *et al.*, 2003); consequently, patient-centred care is compromised.

Research comparing GP and nurse practitioner consultation shows that nurse practitioners talked more with their patients than GPs when seeing patients who had requested 'same day' appointments (Seale *et al.*, 2005). Other studies revealed that patients who consulted nurse practitioners were given more information and were generally more satisfied than those who consulted their GPs (Kinnersley *et al.*, 2000). However, such patient-centred care demands more of the professional's time: the length of nurse consultation is generally longer than that of doctor consultation (Kinnersley *et al.*, 2000; Seale *et al.*, 2005). Time is costly, and thus there is pressure for nurses to reduce their consultation time (Seale *et al.*, 2005). In addition, as nurses increasingly expand their role, focusing on patients' medical problems and working more like doctors, they run the risk of undermining their traditional identity of holism and personal care (Charles-Jones *et al.*, 2003).

Conclusions

This overview of partnership working in the UK health setting projects a complex picture. Despite partnership being central to the UK government's public service policy objectives, there is no consensus in the definition and no agreement of the characteristics of partnership working (McLaughlin, 2004; Wildridge *et al.*, 2004). The development of partnership working is therefore left to local interpretation. Furthermore, there are inconsistencies in successive government policy that challenge partnership working. The requirements of organisations to drive down costs with competitive tendering negate the building of relationships based on trust (Hudson and Henwood, 2002).

Nonetheless, there is evidence of slow progress at both organisational and professional levels. These achievements have been possible because of the commitment of individuals who have worked hard to remove the barriers created by past historical relationships (English, 1997; Benson, 2005).

Partnership is often promoted as a positive development (Department of Health, 1997). This review demonstrates that at all levels partnership has both positive and negative effects. The positive outcomes include improved working relationships and pooling of expertise; most importantly, partnership between professionals and patients helps to deliver a patient-focused service (McLaughlin, 2004). However, it is important to recognise the barriers to successful partnership working: the historical health and social care divide; the competitive culture created by tendering and league tables; and the tradition of uni-professional training. Partnership working requires a facilitative legislative framework and a commitment and willingness to work together. Moreover, policy makers must accept that partnership working, which is about building relationships based on trust and understanding, takes time.

The human and financial costs of partnership working should be acknowledged if an appropriate level of support is to be made available. It is too easy to assume that the sharing of resources, including expertise, will reduce costs. Such assumptions must be tested if partnership working is to be sustained on a long-term basis. All interested parties must recognise that during the transition, partnership development will set back services while organisations work through the changes (Fulop *et al.*, 2002) and staff develop interpersonal trust (Macdonald and Chrisp, 2005).

Part 2
An overview of partnership in psychiatric care services
Peter J. Martin

Intention

- To examine 'partnership' within a psychiatric setting.
- To outline how relationships in psychiatry affect 'partnership'.

Introduction

Partnership is a strategic and operational ambition throughout the UK health system. Those who work within these services are expected to formulate partnerships between individuals and health care workers as well as between statutory and non-statutory services. The term *partnership* is used with a lack of clarity in relation to its meaning and in how it may be delivered in a psychiatric context. Within the psychiatric services partnership may be a goal that is unattainable as a consequence of fundamental complications in the context in which it is employed.

Partnership?

As the previous paper by Eldridge noted, there is no universally accepted definition of partnership as it is currently used in health and social services. The word is used, in its broadest sense, to imply work undertaken by two or more people toward common goals. The literature abounds with examples of the word *part-*

nership within a psychiatric context, for example Department of Health (2001a, 2004, 2005b), Nursing and Midwifery Council (2004) and Sainsbury Centre for Mental Health (2006). These documents all use partnership as a positive and significant component of psychiatric services, but do not consistently apply the term.

There are several terms that describe the structured relationship between service users and service providers. Through the 'working alliance' or 'therapeutic relationship', health care professionals engage service users in a manner that leads to mutually beneficial outcomes. These terms are applied in a formal therapeutic sense and recognise that the relationship is professional with clearly demarcated parameters. Whilst similarities in the relationship are apparent between these two terms and 'partnership', such boundaries have not been delineated in partnership working. Barker suggests that the term *alliance* might be used in preference to partnership. 'Alliance' accepts that the parties involved have differing motives and power bases, but pursue shared goals (Barker, 1999a). Similarly, the term *collaborative working* is used to describe the way service providers work together. The term implies that current circumstances make collaborative working mutually advantageous.

Partnership between service users and service providers

There is an absence of literature about partnership written from a user perspective and much of the available literature on partnerships fails to consider the potentially negative aspects of partnership working (National Institute for Mental Health in England, 2003a). The use of the term *service user* may, in itself, be problematic to defining partnership within psychiatry. A service user has a need that is provided for by service providers; this does not suggest a relationship that is mutually beneficial or based on equality, as would be anticipated within a partnership.

The needs of the individual service user in the psychiatric services are unique. Providing treatment for presenting symptoms is ineffective unless the complex and interrelated physical, psychological and social needs of the person are tackled simultaneously. The social world is a 'sleeping' partner within the partnership between service user and service provider and impacts upon the goals of each in different ways. For the service user the social world may be the root of the perceived problem; for the service provider, the social world may dictate which goals can and cannot be achieved.

There is a difficult balance to be struck between the risk and vulnerability of people with mental health needs (National Institute for Mental Health in England, 2003a). Despite education and awareness campaigns, the public continue to perceive violence and mental illness to be synonymous. There is irrefutable evidence that people with histories of mental illness have harmed others (Royal College of Psychiatrists, 1996); however, the incidence remains less commonplace than assault by persons not considered mentally ill (Department of Health, 2001b). Each time a service user exhibits violence to self or others services appear to become more custodial and less therapeutic, with greater emphasis on the management of risk and less on the needs of the individual. Media and related socio-political pressures stimulate an increasingly traditional paternalistic concept of care (Barker, 1999b). Health care professionals exercise power over the individual when the needs of society and the needs of the individual are in conflict; it is difficult to establish a partnership in such circumstances.

The current review (Department of Health, 2005b) of mental health nursing seeks to answer the question: *'How can mental health nursing best contribute to the care of service users in the future?'* The summary of responses to the consultation (Department of Health, 2006b) identified that there was a need to strengthen partnerships with service users and empower them. Strengthening partnerships was seen as 'central to effective risk assessment and management' (Department of Health, 2006b, p. 6). The relationship with service users in states of acute distress is problematic in terms of partnership. Psychiatric nurses may find themselves in a dilemma with regard to the goal of the partnership. The goal of the service users may be 'freedom', whilst the goals of the community may be 'containment'. The psychiatric nurse must maintain optimum safety for all, which may be at the expense of curtailing the freedom of the individual with whom he is in 'partnership'.

The impact of the social world can also be seen within professional power. The authority of health care professionals is derived from, and is influenced by, the values of society in relation to perceptions of sanity and madness. Psychiatric practice requires 'sane' health care professionals to make decisions, based upon professional knowledge and competence (Eraut, 1994), about the 'sanity' of service users. From the perspective of the user, these decisions present a powerful message that they are unacceptable to society: bad and powerless (Champ, 1999). Psychiatric nurses should seek, amongst other things, to prevent, or at least limit, the damage caused by the abuse of trust and power experienced by psychiatric service users (Davidson, 1998).

The most fundamental demonstration of power within the psychiatric services is the use by health care workers of legislation to force individuals into containment and treatment. Such activity is incompatible with equity and trust in a partnership-based relationship. New mental health legislation proposes a fundamental rethinking of how the law can be used in mental health services with due consideration to other legislation such as the Human Rights Act (1998). The government announced legislation in July 1998 (Department of Health, 1999c) that attempts to make mental health law compatible with contemporary mental health care. *Reforming the Mental Health Act* (Department of Health, 2000b) puts forward the Government's proposals for legislation in the form of a consultation. At the time of writing no consensus has been achieved in relation to the form of the new act and consultation continues. However, the initial proposals put forward by the Government have generated considerable antipathy from service user groups and the health and legal professions alike. A primary objection to the legislation is how power will be exercised over service users within the community by mental health professionals.

Carers should, where appropriate, also be a component of partnerships. The current framework for the support of carers by service providers has been outlined in the NSF Standard 6 (Department of Health, 1999c). This standard recognises that a significant proportion of those with mental illness receive care from 'informal' carers. Providing help, advice and services to these carers is a good way of ensuring that people with mental illness receive the support that they require (Department of Health, 1999c). Recognising the essential contribution that carers make to the psychiatric service and providing appropriate support is crucial. However, it adds a further dimension to partnership within psychiatry where the aims of the carer, the service user and the health care professional may be in conflict. The unequal distribution of power within the psychiatric services may lead to service users being the least powerful component of the partnership.

Psychiatric nurses have many strong voices that have helped, and are helping, to maintain a clear vision of the role and work of the psychiatric nurse. Foremost of these voices are Peplau and Barker. Peplau's contribution to mental health nursing was to ground practice within the interpersonal relationship (Peplau, 1988); her work still resonates with the everyday problems of practice encountered by psychiatric nurses. Peplau's description of the changing aspects of nurse–patient relations, presented as a continuum (Peplau, 1988), has relevance to the debate about partnership. Peplau notes that at the first encounter between patient and nurse, whom she describes as 'strangers', each has entirely separate goals and interests. At the other end of the continuum the nurse and the patient engage in a collaborative effort to solve a problem productively and together. As the nurse and patient move along this continuum mutual understanding of the role grows and the actions required of both parties to solve the problem become apparent. This requires nurse and patient to work together, but as discrete collaborators; the concern is the function of common understanding and shared endeavour within the relationship. Such functions may, in contemporary writing, be described as partnership, but such contemporary writings appear to present 'partnership' as the goal itself. Peplau recognises the existence of conflicting goals and recognises it as an area where nurses can aid patients to vary their goals in line with what is possible (Peplau, 1988, p. 97):

Nursing goals are often obstacles to the patient's goals; communicating in the interpersonal relationship aids both the nurse and the patient to clarify their goals and to reach common understanding.

Barker and Buchanan-Barker's Tidal Model outlines a model of psychiatric services which is empowering with a strong emphasis on *caring with* rather than *caring for* or *caring about* (Barker and Buchanan-Barker, 2005, p. 23). Like Peplau, Barker and Buchanan-Barker recognise that risk is present in mental health work and conflict will arise between the expressed needs of the service users and their safety, which would compromise partnership. The emphasis at all times remains on the service user, and strategies are provided through the multi-layered structure of care comprising core care plans, security plans and multi-professional teamwork (Barker and Buchanan-Barker, 2005). Barker, as has been noted, rejects partnership in favour of alliance. The relationship between service user and health care worker is crucial to the delivery of psychiatric nursing, but it is a professional therapeutic relationship, not a partnership.

Peplau and Barker's work is underpinned by interpersonal relations, as are partnerships; but the two are not synonymous. Partnership is problematic in terms of understanding what it means and how it can be enacted in a service that is so beset by inequality and power imbalance. Barker (1999) asks:

> Who among us would enter into a 'partnership' with someone who might choose, or be required, to use the power of the law against us should we decide to disagree with his or her worldview?

The relationship between the individual and the services/service representatives is problematic. It is a relationship that is far from equal and partnership may not be a realistic aspiration with the inherent risk of tokenism.

Partnership between service providers

Establishing partnership between the various components of the psychiatric services is complex. However, it is seen as a 'must do' for mental health services for a range of political, financial and practical reasons (Sainsbury Centre for Mental Health, 2000) and should be a government priority (National Institute for Mental Health in England, 2003b). Yet there are substantial barriers to partnership working and services need to work at developing partnership arrangements in order to demonstrate good practice.

New service components

Psychiatric services in the UK have been in a state of transition for the past fifty years; the pace of change and development has been particularly notable in the last two decades (Sainsbury Centre for Mental Health, 2005). The latter part of the 1990s saw the closure of many of the large psychiatric institutions which represented a significant shift in the focus of service provision from an institutional to community-based care service. Whilst in transition this shift appeared to be the goal in itself from which service stability would follow. However, services are now in a state of continuous evolution or redevelopment. Traditional partnerships that existed within the large institutions have been fractured. Service providers have had to review ways of working and thinking about how services are constructed to enable partnerships to be developed and to work effectively. Intra-organisation working has been reviewed to manage the decrease in face-to-face communication associated with dispersed community services. In order to develop inter-organisational partnerships different, and often dissimilar providers of mental health services in the community have had to come together to learn about one another and communicate in order to find common ground amongst their service goals. Communication between these service components is essential if service users are to experience improvements in care. The rapid pace of change and service development is challenging and new services take time to become established (National Institute for Mental Health in England, 2003a). In the interim there is a risk that service users may experience fractured rather than seamless services.

Partnerships across professional and organisational divides

There are many factors within organisational structures that obstruct the development of partnerships. Not least is the number of statutory and non-statutory organisations working independently and collaboratively to provide psychiatric care. These organisations operate from differing strategic and operational policies. Mental health charities such as Mind, Sane and Rethink all provide vital components of services available to service users. However, these organisations work differently from each other and from local NHS providers.

Problems in the development of partnerships may not always be apparent at a philosophical level; often partnerships are hampered by mundane problems such as sharing information, risk assessment (e.g. Hancock *et al.*, 1997; Warner *et al.*, 1998; Sainsbury Centre for Mental Health, 2000). Creating new team bases and services within local communities is a simple 'bricks and mortar' task, changing the culture within organisations is far more problematic and time-consuming. These problems, brought about by disparate perspectives, could be resolved by the establishment of a single set of competencies and values and a real commitment to involvement at an organisational and community level to learn how to get the practicalities right (Sainsbury Centre for Mental Health, 2000; National Institute for Mental Health in England, 2003a).

Communication problems between statutory and non-statutory components of psychiatric service with different practice ideologies have led to the creation of a list of common competencies. *The Ten Essential Shared Capabilities* published by the Department of Health (2004) is described as 'best practice guidance'. The document attempts to create a competency framework for the whole mental health workforce. Working with service users in partnership is the first of the ten listed capabilities (Department of Health, 2004, p. 3).

> Working in partnership. Developing and maintaining constructive working relationships with service users, carers, families, colleagues, lay people and wider community networks. Working positively with any tensions created by conflicts of interest or aspiration that may arise between the partners in care.

In *The Ten Essential Shared Capabilities* it is argued that service users should be viewed as partners rather than passive recipients of care; this may require the worker to be 'assertive in their engagement' (Department of Health, 2004, Appendix D). The involvement of the service user in the partnership is described as a requirement of the professional and not necessarily perceived as desirable and useful by the service user. Active involvement by service users in, and commitment to, a care plan developed with professionals is desirable; whether this can be said to be a partnership is a very different matter.

Professional guidance

Establishing partnerships across professional groups for the benefit of service users is often problematic. Professional groups within psychiatry, such as psychiatrists, nurses, social workers and occupational therapists, often hold divergent views about mental illness that shape professional understanding of psychiatric care: for example, psychodynamic, behavioural, social and disease (see Tyrer and Steinberg, 1999). This is less of an issue within general health care, where there is little dispute about the source of the problem in, for example, cardiac arrest. In psychiatry, the understanding of the source of the problem (such as an eating disorder) may impact upon the choice of treatment options. These differing perspectives create conflict and communication problems between professional groups.

Partnership, as promulgated by professional and regulatory bodies within nursing, also presents a particular perspective that appears to emphasise the desirability of partnership without providing a clear definition of the term. The Royal College of Nursing (2003) produced a definition of nursing which stated:

> A commitment to partnership – Nurses work in partnership with patients, their relatives and other carers, and in collaboration with others as members of a multi-disciplinary team....

Similarly, the Nursing and Midwifery Council Code of Professional Conduct (2004) states:

> 2.1 You must recognise and respect the role of patients and clients as partners in their care and the contribution they can make to it. This involves identifying their preferences regarding care and respecting these within the limits of professional practice, existing legislation, resources and the goals of the therapeutic relationship.

The Royal College of Nursing and Nursing and Midwifery Council use partnership to underpin the professional role of the nurse. The Royal College of Nursing definition, 'a commitment to partnership', is an unambiguous statement. This commitment is not mediated by any other factors with which a psychiatric nurse may be confronted. The Nursing and Midwifery Council definition limits the scope of the partnership between service user and service provider by using the term 'within the limits'. The obligation is placed on the nurse to work within professional practice, legislation resources and goals of the therapeutic relationship.

Conclusion

Partnership is both a strategic vision and an operational model of practice. As a service vision, partnership is a prototypical form of service in which participants work together in harmony to attain a shared goal. As an operational model of practice, partnership seeks to be inclusive in attaining goals that are a pragmatic compromise for participants with different aspirations and power resources. The complexity and power imbalances within contemporary psychiatric services make it unlikely that partnership may be anything other than a service vision.

This paper has posed some challenges to the concept of partnership within a psychiatric setting. In the following chapters different forms of partnership will be presented and discussed. In the concluding section of this book reflection on these papers may provide some indicators for the development of good practice within psychiatric and mental health nursing.

References

Anthony-Pillai, R. (2004) Man wins battle to keep receiving life support Man wins battle to keep receiving life support: doctors must always give patients best possible care. *British Medical Journal*, **329** (7464), 515.

Association of the British Pharmaceutical Industry (1999) *The Expert Patient Survey*. ABPI, London. (http://www.abpi.org.uk/publications/publication_details/expert_patient/survey.asp; Last accessed 14 February 2006)

Audit Commission (1995) *For Your Information – A Study of Information Management and Systems in the Acute Hospital*. HMSO, London.

Barker, P. (1999a) *The Philosophy and Practice of Psychiatric Nursing*. Churchill Livingstone, Edinburgh.

Barker, P. (1999b) What are psychiatric nurses needed for? Developing a theory of essential nursing practice. *Journal of Psychiatric and Mental Health Nursing*, **6**, 273–82.

Barker, P. and Buchanan-Barker, P. (2005) *The Tidal Model*. Brunner-Routledge, Hove.

Barlow, J. H., Turner, A. P. and Wright, C. (2000) A randomised controlled study of the arthritis self-management programme in the UK. *Heath Education Research*, **15**, 665–80.

Benson, L. (2005) Working with a nurse called 'Dr'. *GP*, 14 October, p. 41.

Britten, N. (1994) Patients' ideas about medicines: a qualitative study in a general practice population. *British Journal of General Practice*, **44**, 465–8.

Campion, P., Foulkes, J., Neighbour, R. and Tate, P. (2002) Patient centredness in the MRCGP video examination: analysis of large cohort. *British Medical Journal*, **325**, 691–2.

Champ, S. (1999) A most precious thread. In: *From the Ashes of Experience* (eds. P. Barker, P. Campbell and B. Davidson). Whurr, London.

Charles, C., Whelan, T. and Gafni, A. (1999) What do we mean by partnership in making decisions about treatment? *British Medical Journal*, **319**, 780–2.

Charles-Jones, H., Latimer, J. and May, C. (2003) Transforming general practice: the redistribution of medical work in primary care. *Sociology of Health and Illness*, **25**(1), 71–92.

Charlesworth, J. (2001) Negotiating and managing partnership in primary care. *Health and Social Care in the Community*, **9**(5), 279–85.

Clark, J. and Glendinning, C. (2002) Partnership and the remaking of welfare governance. In: *Partnership, New Labour and Governance of Welfare* (eds. C. Glendinning, M. Powell and K. Rummery). Policy Press, Bristol.

Clinical Systems Group (1998) *Improving Clinical Communications*. NHS Executive, London.

Coleman, A. and Rummery, K. (2003) Social services representation in primary care groups and trusts. *Journal of Inter-Professional Care*, **17**(3), 273–80.

Connect (2000) Ten statements about concordance. *Connect*, **6**, 2–3.

Davidson, B. (1998) The role of the psychiatric nurse. In: *Psychiatric Nursing Ethical Strife* (eds. P. Barker and B. Davidson). Edward Arnold, London.

Denner, S. (1995) Extending professional practice: benefits and pitfalls. *Nursing Times*, **91**(14), 27–9.

Department of Health (1997) *The New NHS: Modern, Dependable*. Department of Health, London.

Department of Health (1999a) *Nurses, Midwife and Health Visitor Consultants: Establishing Posts and Making Appointments*. Health Service Circular 1999/217. NHS Executive, Leeds.

Department of Health (1999b) *Our Healthier Nation: Saving Lives*. The Stationery Office, London.

Department of Health (1999c) *National Service Frameworks – Mental Health*. Department of Health, London.

Department of Health (2000a) *The NHS Plan: A Plan for Investment, a Plan for Reform*. Department of Health, London.

Department of Health (2000b) *Reforming the Mental Health Act*. Department of Health, London.

Department of Health (2001a) *The Journey to Recovery – the Government's Vision for Mental Health Care*. Department of Health, London.

Department of Health (2001b) *Safety First – 5 Year Report of the National Confidential Inquiry Into Suicide and Homicide by People with Mental Illness*. Department of Health, London.

Department of Health (2004) *The Ten Essential Shared Capabilities*. Department of Health, London.

Department of Health (2005a) *Commissioning a Patient-led NHS*. Gateway Reference No 5312. Department of Health, London.

Department of Health (2005b) *Chief Nursing Officer's Review of Mental Health Nursing*. Department of Health, London.

Department of Health (2006a) *Best Practice: Examples of Common Learning and Inter-professional Education from Modernising Allied Health Profes-*

sionals Education First Wave Sites. Department of Health, London (http://www.dh.gov.uk/PolicyAndGuidance/HumanResourcesAndTraining/LearningAndPersonalDevelopment/PreRegistration/PreRegistrationArticle/fs/en?CONTENT_ID=4031544&chk=gDXovL; Last accessed 14 February 2006)

Department of Health (2006b) *Chief Nursing Officer's Review of Mental Health Nursing – Summary of Responses to the Consultation*. Department of Health, London.

Dowling, S., Martin, R., Skidmore, P., Doyal, L., Cameron, A. and Lloyd, S. (1996) Nurses taking on junior doctors' work: a confusion of accountability. *British Medical Journal*, **312**, 1211–14.

Dowrick, C., May, C., Richardson, M. and Bundred, P. (1996) The bio-psychosocial model of general practice: rhetoric or reality? *British Journal of General Practice*, **46**, 105–7.

Dyer, C. (2005) Parent fails to overturn ruling not to resuscitate baby. *British Medical Journal*, **330**, 985.

Easen, P., Atkins, M. and Dyson, A. (2000) Inter-professional collaboration and conceptualisation of practice. *Children and Society*, **14**, 355–67.

Eldridge, K. and Ramkhelawon, K. (1999) *Implementing Unified Case Notes – Interim Report to the Four London NHS Trusts*. University of Essex, Colchester.

English, T. (1997) Personal paper: medicine in the 1990s needs a team approach. *British Medical Journal*, **314**, 661.

Eraut, M. (1994) *Developing Professional Knowledge and Competence*. Routledge Falmer, London:

Frank, A. W. (2002) Relations of caring: demoralisation and remoralisation in the clinic. *International Journal for Human Caring*, **6**(2), 13–19.

Freeth, D. (2001) Sustaining inter-professional collaboration. *Journal of Inter-professional Care*, **15**(1), 37–46.

Fulop, N., Protopsaltis, G., Hutchings, A., King, A., Allen, P., Normand, C. and Walters, R. (2002) Process and act of mergers of NHS trusts: multi-centre case study and management cost analysis. *British Medical Journal*, **325**, 246.

Garside, P. (1999) Evidence based merger? *British Medical Journal*, **318**, 345–6.

Gould, M. (2004) Merger pressures on primary care trusts threatened to blur local focus. *Health Service Journal*, **114**, 10–11.

Hancock, M., Vilneau, L. and Hill, R. (1997) *Together We Stand*. Sainsbury Centre for Mental Health, London.

Hardy, B., Hudson, B. and Waddington, E. (2000) *What Makes a Good Partnership? A Partnership Assessment Tool*. Nuffield Institute for Health, Leeds.

Health Service Ombudsman for England (1998) *Investigations of Complaints About Clinical Failings – Full Text of Selected Cases*. Case no: E.1422/97-98 – Insufficient assessment and monitoring by nursing and medical staff, and inadequate care (http://www.ombudsman.org.uk/improving_services/special_reports/hsc/clinical_failings/failings_E1422_full_apB.html; last accessed 14 February 2006).

Health Service Ombudsman for England (2001) *Selected Investigations Completed December 2000–March 2001 Part II*. Case no: E.1777/99-00 – Failure to diagnose and treat a patient with septicaemia; communication between staff; and inadequate response to recommendations of an independent panel (http://www.ombudsman.org.uk/improving_services/selected_cases/HSC/ic0103/pt2-e1777.html; last accessed 17/02/2006).

Health Service Ombudsman for England (2002) *Selected Investigations Completed April–July 2002*. Case no: E.215/00-01 – Poor care and treatment, record-keeping, communication and complaint handling (http://www.ombudsman.org.uk/improving_services/selected_cases/HSC/ic0206/pt2-e215.html; last accessed 14 February 2006).

Heath, I. (2003) A wolf in sheep's clothing: a critical look at the ethics of drug taking. *British Medical Journal*, **327**, 856–8.

Hewison, A. (1995) Nurses' power in interactions with patients. *Journal of Advanced Nursing*, **21**, 75–82.

Hudson, B. and Henwood, M. (2002) The NHS and social care: the final countdown? *Policy and Politics*, **30**(2), 153–66.

Human Rights Act (1998) http://www.opsi.gov.uk/ACTS/acts1998/19980042.htm.

Jorm, C. and Kam, P. (2004) Does medical culture limit doctors' adoption of quality improvement? Lesson from Camelot. *Journal of Health Service Research Policy*, **9**(4), 248–51.

Kelly, M. (2001) *The Cancer Collaborative Services Project*. Colorectal Disease, **4**, 365–6.

Kennedy, A., Gask, L. and Rogers, A. (2005) Training professionals to engage with and promote self-management. *Health Education Research – Theory and Practice*, **20**(5), 567–78.

Kennedy, I. (2001) *Learning from Bristol – the Report of the Public Enquiry into Children's Heart Surgery at the Bristol Royal Infirmary 1984–1995*. Department of Health, London.

Kinnersley, P., Anderson, E., Parry, K., Clement, J., Stainthorpe, A., Fraser, A., Butler, C. and Rogers, C. (2000) Randomised control trial of nurse practitioner versus general practitioner care for patients requesting 'same day' consultation in primary care. *British Medical Journal*, **320**, 1043–8.

Laidler, P. (1994) *Stroke Rehabilitation – Structure and Strategy*. Chapman & Hall, London.

Lorig, K., Sobel, D., Stewart, A., Brown, B., Bandura, A. and Ritter, P. (1999) Evidence suggesting that a chronic disease self management programme can improve health status while reducing hospitalisation. A randomised control trial. *Medical Care*, **37**, 5–14.

Lowndes, V., Nanton, A., McCabe, C. and Skelcher, C. (1997) Networks, partnerships and urban regeneration. *Local Economy*, **11**(4), 333–42.

Macdonald, S. and Chrisp, T. (2005) Acknowledging the purposes of partnership. *Journal of Business Ethics*, **59**(4), 307–17.

MacGregor, S. (1998) From paternalism to partnership. *British Medical Journal*, **317**, 221.

Mackay, L. (1993) *Conflicts in Care: Medicine and Nursing*. Chapman & Hall, London.

May, C., Dowrick, C. and Richardson, M. (1996) The confidential patient: the social construction of therapeutic relationships in general medical practice. *Sociological Review*, **44**(2), 187–203.

Marinker, M. and Shaw, J. (2003) Not to be taken as directed. *British Medical Journal*, **326**, 348–9.

Mariotto, A. (1999) Patient partnership is not a magic formula. *British Medical Journal*, **319**, 783.

McLaughlin, H. (2004) Partnership: panacea or pretence? *Journal of Interprofessional Care*, **18**(2), 103–13.

National Confidential Enquiry into Peri-Operative Deaths (2002) *Functioning as a Team? The 2002 Report of the National Confidential Enquiry into Perioperative Deaths*. National Confidential Enquiry into Peri-Operative Deaths, London.

National Institute for Mental Health in England (2003a) *Cases for Change: a Review of the Foundations of Mental Health Policy and Practice 1997–2002 – Introduction*. National Institute for Mental Health in England, Leeds.

National Institute for Mental Health in England (2003b) *Cases for Change: A Review of the Foundations of Mental Health Policy and Practice 1997–2002 – Partnership Working Across Health and Social Care*. National Institute for Mental Health in England, Leeds.

NHS Centre for Review and Dissemination (1997) *Concentration and Choice in the Provision of Hospital Services – CRD Report No 8*. University of York, York.

Nursing and Midwifery Council (2004) *The NMC Code of Professional Conduct: Standards for Conduct, Performance and Ethics*. Nursing and Midwifery Council, London

Ovretveit, J., Mathias, P. and Thompson, T. (eds.) (1997) *Inter-Professional Working for Health and Social Care*. Macmillan, Basingstoke.

Peplau, H. (1988) *Interpersonal Relations in Nursing*. Macmillan, London.

Price, A. and Williams, A. (2003) Primary care nurse practitioners and the interface with secondary care: a qualitative study of referral practice. *Journal of Inter-Professional Care*, **17**(3), 239–50.

Radcliffe, M. (2000) Personal views: doctors and nurses: new game, same result. *British Medical Journal*, **320**, 1085.

Richards, T. (1998) Partnership with patients. *British Medical Journal*, **316**, 85–6.

Richardson, G. and Maynard, A. (1995) *Few Doctors? More Nurses? A Review of the Knowledge Base of Doctor–Nurse Substitution*. Discussion Paper 135, Centre for Health Economics, York Health Economics Consortium, NHS Centre for Review and Dissemination. University of York, York.

Royal College of Nursing (2003) *Defining Nursing*. Royal College of Nursing, London.

Royal College of Psychiatrists (1996) *Report of the Confidential Inquiry into Homicides and Suicides by Mentally Ill People*. Royal College of Psychiatrists, London.

Rumbold, J. M. M. (2004) Media coverage. *British Medical Journal*, **329** (7461), 309.

Rummery, K. (1999) The way forward for joint working? Involving primary care in the commissioning of social care services. *Journal of Inter-Professional Care*, **13**(3), 207–18.

Rummery, K. (2003) Progress towards partnership? The development of relations between primary care organisations and social services concerning older people services in the UK. *Social Policy and Society*, **3**(1), 33–42.

Sainsbury Centre for Mental Health (2000) Taking Your Partners: Using Opportunities for Inter-agency Partnership in Mental Health. Sainsbury Centre for Mental Health, London.

Sainsbury Centre for Mental Health (2005) *Beyond the Water Towers*. Sainsbury Centre for Mental Health, London.

Sainsbury Centre for Mental Health (2006) *The Future of Mental Health: a Vision for 2015*. Sainsbury Centre for Mental Health, London.

Seale, C., Anderson, C. and Kinnersley, P. (2005) Comparison of GP and nurse practitioner consultation: an observational study. *British Journal of General Practice*, **55**, 938–43.

Shaw, J. and Baker, M. (2004) Expert patient – dream or nightmare? *British Medical Journal*, **328**, 723–4.

Sheldon, T. and Maynard, A. (1999) Politicians may not have the same goals as clinicians with regard to mergers. *British Medical Journal*, **318**, 1762.

Smeltzer, C., Hines, P., Beebe, H. and Keller, B. (1996) Streamlining documentation: an opportunity to reduce costs and increase nurse clinicians' time with patients. *Journal of Nursing Care Quarterly*, **10**(4), 66–77.

Smith, R. (2003) Preparing for partnership. *British Medical Journal*, **326**, 7402.

Stein, L. (1967) The doctor–nurse game. *Archives of General Psychiatry*, **16**(6), 699–703.

Stein, L., Watts, D. T., and Howell, T. (1990) The doctor–nurse game revisited. *New England Journal of Medicine*, **322**(8), 546–9.

Sweet, S. and Norman, I. (1995) The nurse–doctor relationship: a selective literature review. *Journal of Advanced Nursing*, **22**, 165–70.

Tailby, S., Richardson, M., Stewart, P., Danford, A. and Upchurch, M. (2004) Partnership at work and worker participation: an NHS case study. *Industrial Relations Journal*, **35**(5), 403–18.

Taylor, M. (2000) Patient care (empowerment): a local view. *British Medical Journal*, **320**, 1663–4.

The Times (2004) Incompatibility of GMC life prolonging guidelines. *The Times*, 10 August, p. 37.

Tomlinson, F. (2005) Idealistic and pragmatic version of the discourse of partnership. *Organisation Studies*, **26**(8), 1169–88.

Tyrer, P. and Steinberg, D. (1999) *Models for Mental Disorder*, 3rd edn. John Wiley & Sons, Chichester.

Walsh, K., Smith, J., Dixon, J., Edwards, N., Hunter, D., Mays, N., Normand, C. and Robinson, R. (2004) Primary care trusts. *British Medical Journal*, **329**, 871–2.

Warner, L., Ford, R., Bagnalls, S., Morgan, S., McDaid, C. and Mawhinney, S. (1998) *Down Your Street*. Sainsbury Centre for Mental Health, London.

White, C. (2003) Doctors fail to grasp concept of concordance. *British Medical Journal*, **327**, 642.

Wildridge, V., Childs, S., Cawthra, L. and Madge, B. (2004) How to create successful partnerships – a review of the literature. *Health Information and Libraries Journal*, **21**, 3–19.

Williams, A., Robins, T. and Sibbald, B. (1997) *Cultural Differences Between Medicine and Nursing: Implications for Primary Care. A Summary Report.* National Primary Care Research and Development Centre, Manchester.

Wilson, P. (2001) A policy analysis of the expert patient in the United Kingdom: self-care as an expression of pastoral power? *Health and Social Care in the Community*, **9**(3), 134–42.

Woodward, V., Webb, C. and Prowse, M. (2005) Nurse consultants: their characteristics and achievements. *Journal of Clinical Nursing*, **14**, 845–54.

CHAPTER 2

Service users and service providers

Introduction

Kimmy Eldridge

This chapter comprises two research reports and a critical review that extracts common themes relating to partnership working from two studies. The two small-scale research studies were completed as part of a master's degree at the University of Essex:

- 'Engaging quitters, preventing relapse and supporting long-term cessation of smoking' by Diane Treadwell
- 'Living with type II diabetes: do partnerships between patients, family and health care professionals impact upon patients' experience?' by Jane Young

In Treadwell's study, the researcher was a practice nurse who felt that the training she had received to provide level two smoking-cessation programmes had not prepared her adequately to work with relapsed quitters. She did not understand their needs and was not aware of any interventions that have been shown to be beneficial to this particular patient group. A systematic literature review did not provide answers to her questions and gave her justification to design a small-scale exploratory research study.

In Young's study, the researcher, who is a clinical nurse specialist, observed that conversion to insulin led to weight gain. Furthermore, patients reported that they were 'worse off' when receiving insulin than when they were being treated with oral medication. A literature review showed that existing quality-of-life measures tended to focus on the agenda of the researchers rather than that of the patients. Such approaches had not advanced understanding of the real concerns of the patients. The justification for a small-scale exploratory study was thus established.

Part I
Smoking cessation: engaging quitters, preventing relapse and supporting long-term cessation
Diane Treadwell

Intention

■ To examine the experience of individuals who tried to stop their smoking habit and had completed a relapse-prevention programme
■ To identify ways ways through which effective support could be provided to sustain smoking cessation.

Introduction

Smoking killed over 120,000 people in the UK in 1995: 1 in 5 of all deaths, equivalent to 13 people per hour, every hour of every day (Callum, 1998). An estimated four million smokers per year attempt to quit, but only 3–6% succeed (National Institute for Clinical Excellence, 2002).

Evidence shows that smoking-cessation programmes work. Stapleton (2001) states that these programmes and treatments are probably the most cost-effective way in which the National Health Service (NHS) is spending money. However, in order for the patient and society to benefit, lifelong cessation must be the ultimate goal. Relapse rates can be as high as 60%, and few trials have published data of abstinence beyond one year (Stapleton, 1998).

Background

This study stemmed from my awareness as a practice nurse that motivated quitters relapsed back to smoking within one year. However, it was difficult to offer them help in relapse prevention. I was trained to provide level two smoking cessation; this involves counselling and support on a one-to-one basis while a person is attempting to quit smoking, either with or without the addition of pharmaceutical support in the form of either nicotine replacement or Bupropion. However, this training had not adequately prepared me for working with relapsed quitters. I did not feel that I understood their needs or was aware of strategies that had been proven to be of benefit. I therefore felt that more information would benefit both future quitters as well as relapsers.

This research study examined the experience of relapse from the perspective of patients who had undergone a recognised programme of smoking cessation.

Key literature review

In 2000, around 170 new papers were published each month in the field of smoking cessation (West *et al.*, 2000). My literature search, using the Cinahl, PubMed, Medline and Ovid databases, retrieved over 1000 citations containing the words 'smoking cessation' alone, but only 56 containing 'smoking cessation' and 'relapse' together. The work dates from 1980 to 2003, with the older work focusing on relapse and the newer work examining smoking-cessation programmes.

The majority of the literature discussed relapse in relation to postpartum women, and therefore the data cannot be generalised. There was a distinct lack of data about relapse among general populations. Scotts *et al.* (1996) make a distinction between pregnant smokers and non-pregnant smokers, stating that pregnant smokers do not go through the same behavioural change process as non-pregnant smokers and that abstinence in pregnancy should be referred to as 'stopping' rather than 'quitting', stopping being a short-term abstinence motivated by an external factor (the baby), thus explaining the high relapse rate in pregnant quitters. Quitting is a long-term cessation and is more associated with internal, intentional processes of change.

Other researchers hold the view that rather than concentrating on trying to prevent relapse, smoking prevalence would be better reduced by targeting large numbers with brief intervention and specialist smoking-cessation programmes combining both behavioural and pharmaceutical support (Curry and McBride, 1994; Niaura *et al.*, 1999; Jarvis, 2002).

Smoking-cessation programmes are relatively effective, but relapse remains high (Leventhal and Cleary, 1980; Schachter, 1982; Brandon *et al.*, 2000). Relapse rates in smokers are estimated at around 40–60% (Stapleton, 1998), with a risk of relapse even after one year of abstinence (Brandon *et al.*, 2000; Krall *et al.*, 2002). Some of the literature suggests relapse occurs because of internal factors such as lack of will power and the lack of self-efficacy, especially in highly tempting and negative situations (e.g. out socialising with friends or when upset), rather than external factors (e.g. lack of support from family) (Curry *et al.*, 1990; Garcia *et al.*, 1990). Bandura (1977, p. 193) defines self-efficacy as 'conviction that one can successfully execute the behaviour required to produce the [desired] outcomes'. Curry *et al.* (1990) discuss motivation for smoking cessation in terms of intrinsic influences (e.g. concerns about negative health consequences) and extrinsic influences (e.g. constant nagging about smoking by spouse).

Individuals that attribute cessation to external factors may be less able to maintain cessation, and this is known as the attribution theory (Prochaska and Di Clemente, 1983; Harackiewicz *et al.*, 1987; Ogden, 2000). This is certainly true of relapsers returning to clinic whose relapse occurred as soon as the course of nicotine replacement therapy (NRT) or Bupropion (Zyban) ended, with some patients stating that relapse was a result of not getting an appointment to see the nurse or doctor. They attributed their quit success to the support of the professional and the use of pharmaceutical intervention (extrinsic motivation).

High relapse rates can be the result of the addictiveness of nicotine and withdrawal symptoms associated with nicotine abstinence. The most effective adjunctive treatment is NRT, but even when cessation continues for several months, relapse risk remains high (Stapleton, 1998). Relapse also occurs long after the withdrawal effect has resolved, and therefore controlling withdrawal effect with NRT or Bupropion (Zyban) is not sufficient to prevent relapse (Royal College of Physicians, 2000).

Reports suggest that there is no clear evidence to demonstrate the effectiveness of relapse prevention (Haaga *et al.*, 1993; West *et al.*, 2003b). Haaga *et al.* (1993) state this may be because of a disagreement between theory and what ex-smokers actually believe to be the reason for relapse. The Government recognises that smokers have a choice (Department of Health, 1999a), a sentiment echoed by Rollnick *et al.* (2000). The Government also states that smokers should exercise this choice in full knowledge of the risks of smoking and passive smoking to their health and the health of others (Department of Health, 1999a).

Smokers should be made aware of the benefits of quitting and the help that is available to assist them (Department of Health 1999a). Current smoking-cessation policy emerged following the publication of *Smoking Kills* (Department of Health, 1999s) and the *Smoking Cessation Guidelines for Health Care Professionals* (West *et al.*, 1998). These guidelines were based on the evidence provided by the Cochrane Collaboration Tobacco Addiction Review Group (http://www.cochrane.org/index0.htm). Up to date information from the Tobacco Addiction Review Group can be accessed via the Cochrane Library, Oxford.

The study

This is a qualitative study, exploring the complex relationship between smoking and relapse, using semi-structured interviews to collect data from seven 'relapsed smokers'. Five were female and two were male. The mean age of respondents was 52 years, ranging from 37 to 67 years.

Non-probability sampling was used in order to identify and recruit a group of 'experts' to the study, who in turn would enable me to explore and understand the lived experiences of relapsed smokers. The respondents were chosen because of their knowledge and experience of smoking cessation, relapse and willingness to participate.

Ethical approval was sought from and granted by the Local Research Ethics Committee. Interviews were taped and the tapes transcribed verbatim. Four interviews took place in the respondents' own homes and three at the respondents' places of work, as this was more convenient for them. Each interview lasted around three-quarters of an hour and all respondents were assured anonymity and confidentiality.

Findings

The findings of this study are compared with the information in the literature in an attempt better to inform practice. The themes identified in the study were:

- Addiction/habit and failure of medication
- Motivation and beliefs (personal, familial and societal)
- The nurse–patient relationship
- Anxiety, stress, boredom
- Enjoyment of smoking
- Health beliefs
- Repeated quit attempts
- Control

The themes were identified by thematic analysis using a grounded theory approach.

These themes have been identified in previous studies of smoking and relapse, which provides support for the trustworthiness of the study (Butler *et al.*, 1998; Bottorf *et al.*, 2000; Wiltshire *et al.*, 2003). The main theme to be discussed in this work will be around the nurse–patient relationship.

Professional conflict, failure of medication

The findings identified the disparity of advice received by patients attending their GP or practice nurse for smoking-cessation advice, despite the professionals all having undergone training in how to provide smoking-cessation support to their patients.

This disparity led to an inequality of service, highlighting the need for recognised training and mentorship programmes for all workers providing a smoking-cessation service. One respondent had received unhelpful advice from a doctor a few years before and so did not feel she would seek advice from a doctor again. She did, however, discuss her breathing and smoking with the practice nurse at her surgery:

> ... [she] mentions my smoking when I go to see her. (*Sharon*)

Nurses and GPs should be encouraged to engage patients and ask them about their smoking status at every opportunity. In the past, GPs were worried that this might damage their relationship with the patient. However, research studies found this not to be the case (Furlow *et al.*, 1996; Butler *et al.*, 1998; West *et al.*, 2000; Sutherland 2003).

Relationships can be damaged if the best smoking-cessation intervention is not matched to the patient or pitched at the right level (Niaura and Abrams, 2002). Getting the right advice and support is not easy. Two of the respondents gave very different ideas about what they wanted from the nurse.

John is a 42-year-old builder and father of two who had not considered quitting smoking until his daughter (aged 4) developed asthma. As a consequence he had taken to smoking outside the house. He himself admitted suffering each year from 'a bad chest' which always got worse in the winter months. He decided this was not helped by his standing outside in all weathers to have his cigarettes. His plan was to quit smoking to help both himself and his daughter. John saw two different nurses at his surgery:

> ... I saw a nurse before ... I went to get the patches and she said don't give up, which I found strange. Christmas and New Year was coming up and she said it was the wrong time to give up. I was in the right frame of mind, but after about three weeks of not smoking, I went to see the nurse and she told me not to stop. I had bought patches and went there to get some more on prescription. She [nurse 1] wanted proof I was going to use them. I was really angry. I went back to ... [nurse 2] after Christmas 'cos I wanted to try again and she got me a prescription for the patches. She phoned to see how I was getting on, but I felt pressured by that. Then I started again. (*John*)

From listening to John it appears that the first nurse did not understand that he had already quit smoking for three weeks before he went to see her. It is difficult to comment having only heard his story, but it is a familiar one. The second nurse probably felt that she was being supportive by making a follow-up call, as there is evidence to suggest that this helps to reduce relapse (Borland *et al.*, 2001).

Brandon *et al.* (2000), however, reported that telephone communication, either alone or in combination with repeated mailings, was ineffective. They found that repeated mailings of *Stay Quit* booklets were significantly more productive in reducing relapse for the year during which they were provided. This relates to John's comment later in the interview:

> I think the nurse should encourage you, but she didn't help me. I don't want the pressure. Without the patches I would never have given up. I felt I was obliged to use the patches because they were doing me a favour by giving them to me. I didn't feel as if they were offering me a service. I felt they begrudged me having them. She [nurse 1] embarrassed me in front of my daughter, which I didn't like. (*John*)

This demonstrates the need to listen and ask what support someone wants; it is then up to the nurse and the patient to come to an understanding about what can be offered and how the quit attempt will proceed. When asked how the nurse could help in the future, John responded:

> Plenty of encouragement, and don't pressurise. Be positive to the patient. I got information from the surgery, but the info with the patches is more helpful than anything. I don't need a lecture from the nurse. (*John*)

In contrast, Bill wanted to be told what to do and when to do it. He felt he would have been more successful had he had more structured involvement from his practice nurse:

> The doctor suggested I see the nurse. I haven't had a quit date given to me. (*Bill*)

When asked if being given a quit date might have helped, he replied:

> Yes, probably. I've had the analyser [*a Smokerlizer which measures the levels of carbon monoxide on the breath of a smoker*]; it's been up and down. Everybody's happy as long as I keep it low. The surgery couldn't set up a programme for me – there was a problem with the computer having set up the appointments for three weeks' time – so it was left to me to phone and book the next appointment. I do as I'm told but I had a couple of things going on at the time, my cholesterol was going through the roof and I had a high BP. I will get there.... (*Bill*)

If it was written down on a piece of paper, what I should do. I'm not a cheating sort of a person. There's no point in cheating, you're cheating yourself not the nurse. I don't care if the nurse tells me off. (*Bill*)

These two exemplars highlight all that is difficult about smoking-cessation intervention and relapse prevention.

Out of the two women who had self-referred, one had experienced a smoking-cessation group programme and the other had attended her practice nurse. Mary, who participated in the group, said:

I started with the smoking cessation thing. It was really good, then I got the patches from the doctor. You have four weeks as a non-smoker then you have nothing, no support. Your motivation is high to start with, then at the four-week stage, it starts to fail. I found it most difficult between weeks 4–6. The group arranged to meet and a few of us turned up.... We needed that extra support. (*Mary*)

When asked what might have helped prevent her from relapsing she said:

... the group going on for longer. Four weeks is just not enough. There was a real group support thing going on.... They were all really helpful, lovely people. The leader is frightening (laughing)... maybe that was enough to prevent us from smoking. I'm not sure about the patches. (*Mary*)

Gill went to her practice nurse when discharged from hospital. She explained:

I went into hospital. I have tried to stop before.... I'll stop for about 4–6 weeks and then just start again.... I got patches from the doctor and also lozenges. Yes I saw the nurse. Only for a few weeks, not long... I can't remember now. The doctor always has a go at me (smiling).... It doesn't help, not really. (*Gill*)

Gill only went to the nurse because the doctor said she must stop. When asked if she thought it might have been different had she decided to go along herself without the doctor referring her, she replied:

I don't know. (*Gill*)

Failure of pharmaceutical support, running out of medication and the inability to get an appointment were also cited as reasons why people smoked:

The patches were worse than the lozenges. The lozenges helped a bit, but the patches were useless. It's completely down to me. It's me that's got to do it. (*Gill*)

I used patches, lozenges and inhalers. The inhalers were OK to start with, but I did get used to them (*Bill*)

When asked why he started smoking again, Bill replied:

I can't think of anything that made me start again. It was just a case of running out of the puffers, so I had a cigarette instead. (*Bill*)

With regard to what might help in the future, Mary talked about the group going on for longer, but said:

I'm not sure about the patches. (*Mary*)

The attribution theory is well documented, and individuals who assign their success to external factors have been found to be less successful (Prochaska and Di Clemente, 1983; Harackiewicz *et al.*, 1987; Ogden, 2000).

Reasons for smoking/relapse

The major factors why people quit smoking are external. Smokers have been made to feel antisocial, deviants and weak. Smoking is looked upon as a waste of money and resources. There is much pressure on smokers from family and friends to quit, and this is enforced by current media campaigns. Health campaigns advertising government and health service provision of help and support to smokers who want to quit also makes smokers vulnerable to public criticism, and if they do not access the support they are seen to not want help.

The fact that people continue to smoke even when confronted with illness related to smoking seems irrational. However, from the study we can deduce that believing health will improve and illness prevented if one stops smoking is low on the agenda as a motivator to quit smoking. People are more likely to quit for others than for themselves. For abstinence to be achieved it is essential that this motivation to quit is internalised. Successful abstinence is dependent on intrinsic reward (Galvin, 1992).

The study showed that most people, when asked, could not specifically say why they relapsed. Enjoyment of smoking featured highly, suggesting that relapse was a consequence of missing that enjoyment. The majority of smokers in the study believed that internal motivation was the key to abstinence, but that they were not motivated in this way. The reason most of them attempted to quit was pressure from family and friends or doctor and or for financial reasons. Lack of willpower and self-motivation were key features in the interviews. However, the respondents did not directly attribute their relapse to lack of willpower or self-motivation.

The major cause of relapse in this study was stress. People began smoking again when they were in highly stressful situations. This finding also translates to my professional experience. Helman (2000) sums this up by calling tobacco a 'chemical comforter'.

There appears to be insufficient evidence out there to support in-depth programmes of relapse prevention and that it would more efficient to focus on supporting the smoker through their quit attempt rather than making additional relapse prevention efforts (Hajek *et al*., 2005).

Recommendations

- **Recommendation 1** Health care workers need to accept that relapse in smoking is a chronic condition and provide support for patients who have experienced this.
- **Recommendation 2** Effective smoking cessation consists of one-to-one or group support, to the right person, at the right time and at the right level. It was evident from the interviews with the two men in the study that individually tailored intervention has a major influence on the response of the patient. Urso (2003) puts forward the 'Five As' (ask, advise, assess, assist and arrange). It is important that individuals take ownership of their quit attempt and that internal motivators for change are identified and nurtured. Patients should be approached about their smoking in a respectful non-judgemental way and professionals should be sensitive to patients' receptivity and treat them as individuals.
- **Recommendation 3** Follow-up appointments should be made during the early stages of the quit process, as it would appear that the early stages are the most vulnerable time.
- **Recommendation 4** Those providing smoking-cessation support must have adequate training. Advisers should select the optimum treatment by learning the efficacy and applicability of all available interventions (Urso, 2003). The Government needs to make recommendations that govern this training (Lennox *et al*., 1998; Gould *et al*., 2000; West *et al*., 2003a).
- **Recommendation 5** In order to prevent relapse, more research needs to be done exploring why relapse occurs. Nurses trained in smoking cessation would be best placed to carry out this type of qualitative study.

Implications

The recommendations are informed by the experiences of relapse smokers as well as the literature. If these recommendations are not adopted, the investment in the current campaign to stop smoking will not achieve the intended outcomes. In addition, there is further risk of alienating smokers through a lack of genuine partnership between professional and smokers.

Conclusion

This was a small scale study with a restricted time-scale and as such has its limitations. From the interviews in this study it can be concluded that the most important aspect of smoking-cessation intervention is a personalised service through partnership; the intervention and follow-up should be tailored to the individual. It is essential to gauge how much support people need and to discuss with them how they would like it delivered, and then plan the support within the constraints of the service.

Part 2
Living with Type II diabetes
Jane Young

Intention

- To examine the lived experience of a group of patients who have progressed from tablet to insulin therapy, and their perception of quality of life on insulin
- To identify the personal cost and benefit effects to the patient.

Introduction

Patient empowerment is central to current health care policy within the arena of chronic disease management (Department of Health, 2001, 2002). Medical opinion accepts and promotes improvement in glycaemic control as the corner-stone of effective diabetic management in patients with Type II diabetes (United Kingdom Prospective Diabetes Study, 1998a). Consequently, patients are con-verted to insulin to reduce the chances of developing diabetes-related complica-tions. However, many patients experience weight gain and an increase in other associated cardiovascular risk factors after the conversion (Douek and Gale, 2001). Some patients have reported that improvement in short-term quality-of-life post-insulin conversion was either minimal or absent (Testa and Simonson, 1998).

This study was designed to gain an understanding of patients' perceptions of issues relating to insulin therapy. The findings were used to improve patients' experience of health care and to build partnership between professionals and patients.

Background

A local audit of 577 patients with Type II diabetes who had attended a district general hospital between January 1999 and October 2002 revealed that those patients converted to insulin therapy had weight gains of between 0.3 kg and 20 kg. Although the latter demonstrates the extreme, the average weight gain of individuals was in excess of 5 kg.

A sub-set of 100 patients taken from this sample demonstrated that 68% of patients showed improvement in their glycaemic control, utilising HbA1c as the means of measurement. HbA1c is a blood test which indicates the amount of glucose that has been absorbed by haemoglobin A1 within the red blood cell over its lifetime and is thus a marker of glycaemic control. Ten per cent of patients enjoyed less favourable control than they had achieved prior to com-mencement of insulin therapy and 8% showed neither improvement nor decline in glycaemic control. The remainder (14%) of this sub-set had not had post-insulin HbA1c measurements performed, thus making it impossible to make comparisons.

Approximately 40 % of the same subset of patients showed a decline in blood pressure control. It should be noted, however, that it cannot be ruled out that the cause of the rise in blood pressure could be linked to natural disease progression in the insulin-resistant Type II patient. It is also not possible to make comparisons of the relationship between weight gain and blood pressure control as a consequence of gaps in the data set. It could be argued that, in some cases, achievement of improvement in glycaemic control is at the expense of the worsening of other cardiovascular risk factors, such as increased weight and blood pressure. This concurs with the findings of Douek and Gale (2001).

Given weight gain and, in some cases, blood pressure increases, this raises the question: What is the personal cost to the patient? Anecdotally some patients had reported feeling worse off on insulin. Walling (2002) argues that patients with Type II diabetes can be switched to insulin without a reduction in their quality of life. However, the author neither alluded to methodology nor how this conclusion was reached.

Key literature review

The review seeks to provide an understanding of the issues that may relate to so-called 'quality of life' in patients with Type II diabetes mellitus. Specifically, it aims to address the following questions:

- What approaches have been used to measure quality of life?
- What impact has insulin therapy had on the quality of life of patients with Type II diabetes mellitus?
- What are the other factors or issues that influence quality of life?

The search for relevant and current literature was conducted using the following key words and phrases: Type II diabetes and insulin, quality of life in diabetes, and living with diabetes. The information sources included Medline (PubMed), Cumulative Index of Nursing and the Allied Health Literature (CINAHL), electronic journal services and the diabetes journals accessed via an initial search utilising the search engine Google. The search focused on the literature published between 1996 and 2003. A hand search was also performed to identify relevant textbooks using the same keywords.

Both the United Kingdom Prospective Diabetes Study (1998a,b) and the Diabetes Control and Complications Trial of 1993 (Zinman, 1997) have provided evidence that focuses on the importance of 'tight' glycaemic control in the battle against the development of both macrovascular and microvascular complications in both Type I and Type II diabetes. It has also been suggested that this primary goal of care should be accompanied by the achievement of a 'relatively normal quality of life' (Rose *et al.*, 2002). However, the difficulty arises in how this conclusion can either be measured or, indeed, achieved. To complicate matters further, the terms health status, quality of life (qol), health-related quality of life (HRqol), well-being, treatment satisfaction and health status are often used interchangeably (Bradley, 2001; Speight, 2002). Furthermore, very little work came to light that reflected quality of life from the patients' perspective.

The difficulty with differentiating health status from quality of life is that impaired health or well-being may lead to, or be, experienced at the same time as impaired quality of life, although this is not always the case. Therefore excellent health does not imply excellent quality of life or vice versa. Well-being, usually defined as a sense of negative or positive well-being or happiness (Pouwer *et al.*, 2001) has been used to measure psychological factors that affect the patient's evaluation of the quality of care they receive (Pouwer *et al.*, 2001). It has also been argued that increased satisfaction and collaboration in the patient–health care professional relationship is associated with better outcomes for patients with diabetes (Ciechanowski *et al.*, 2002). However, it is uncertain who might be the beneficiary: the patient or the health care professional?

The repeated use of scoring systems such as ADDQoL (Audit of Diabetes dependent quality of life) has improved reliability and validity as a means of assessing quality of life (Bradley *et al.*, 2002; Varni *et al.*, 2003). However, the use of quality-of-life measures such as impact profile scores and diabetes symptom check lists shows no statistically significant changes in quality of life parameters (de Grauw *et al.*, 2001).

The study

The aim of the study was to describe the life experiences of patients who receive insulin therapy, rather than to generate specific generalisable quantitative measures. Focus groups were thus chosen as a means of data collection (Bernard 2000; Holloway and Wheeler, 2002; Ritchie and Lewis, 2003). Ethical approval was sought via the Local Research Ethics Committee and the Trust approval was granted via the research and development department.

Twenty-four patients were invited to participate in one of three focus groups. Selection was undertaken to include a spread of age ranges and an equal gender split. Ten female and six male respondents participated in group discussions that lasted one to one and a half hours each. Eight respondents did not attend on the day for a variety of reasons associated with family difficulties, including one patient who was hospitalised on an emergency basis for a non-diabetes-related

Table 2.1 Focus group discussion questions.

▦ What were your immediate thoughts and feelings when you were prescribed insulin and why did you feel that way?

▦ What impact has this had on your quality of life?

▦ Do you feel better on insulin and in what way?

▦ Do you feel worse on insulin and in what way?

▦ Has it affected your weight, the way that you see yourself and your life?

illness. The discussions were taped and later transcribed (see Table 2.1 for focus group discussion questions).

Findings

The following themes emerged from the analysis: physical problems, emotional and family-related problems and reactions to insulin. The overwhelming message that permeates the data collected was one of power and control.

Physical problems

In the majority of cases, patients described negative feelings associated with fear of injections. For example, 'The absolute thought of putting a needle in was horrifying to me personally' and 'I tried to avoid it – my heart dropped'. This reaction for most was short lived: 'I discovered how easy it was' and 'I was quite relieved – no pain'.

Issues relating to weight dominated much of the discussion and emerged fairly early on. This is reflected in the comments: 'I have put on a stone and that is the absolute worse thing that could have happened to me' and 'Since I have been on insulin I have put on 3 stone and now I am struggling to get it off' and 'No-one wants to put on weight'.

Furthermore, this had repercussions for one woman who reported: 'I find myself getting out of breath'.

Other than the correlation between weight gain and insulin resistance (Williams and Pickup, 1999), weight increase appears to have an effect on people's self-esteem and the view that they perceive their family and friends have of them. For example, one woman reported that her husband said 'I can't understand why you are not losing weight'. Most of the respondents felt that this was something over which they had no control and others directed their anger at the health care professional: 'Doctors don't tell you anything' and 'Just be up front about it'.

Problems associated with hypo- and hyperglycaemia caused some concern. In most cases hypoglycaemia was something that the patients feared and which created a feeling that they were not in control: 'I'm always petrified that something is going to happen and I won't get back in time for dinner'.

Hyperglycaemia appeared to be something that caused irritation and was associated with certain types of behaviour such as 'I noticed with high blood sugars that I am really aggressive' and 'You just don't want to do nothing when they are high'. This is substantiated by a study conducted by Koopmanschap (2002), who concluded that hyperglycaemia was negatively associated with quality of life.

Emotional issues and family transactions

The concepts of self-blame and disappointment associated with a sense of failure appeared to be the main reaction to insulin therapy. This was expressed as: 'I was a bit disappointed – I thought that I was doing all right'. This is expanded further in that it became evident that some patients had not come to terms with their diabetes: 'I mean if we all thought about it deep down, it's hard to accept' and 'I wake up in the morning and my sugar levels are normal, which makes me think why am I taking it?'.

Loss of freedom and spontaneity were major issues for most of the respondents and created mixed feelings and perceptions. These can be subdivided into loss of freedom when eating and loss of freedom in more general terms: 'Before I could eat on the hoof' and 'to think that I have to stop and eat when I don't want to' demonstrates frustration with lifestyle changes that were not a matter of personal choice but a necessity of living with diabetes.

In more general terms the impact on quality of life was expressed as 'it's constant – you can't forget it', 'you can't go out all day and you can't do this and you can't do that – it does restrict you', and 'you know that you've got to regulate your life more'. All of these quotations relate to the feeling that the patient did not have control.

The participants also reported the impact of insulin therapy on their family relationships. The necessity to plan the injection and food intake causes tension in personal relationships. As one man reported: 'The biggest inconvenience was to the wife when I went on insulin – I have to inject 20 minutes before a meal. Breakfast is all right, but evening meal – always arguments and a little dig to coincide with the time factor'. This led to the perception that 'I get the feeling in my house that I shouldn't be ill in the first place' and 'I don't think that I have changed, but she does.'

One woman found that her diabetes had became a scapegoat in her relationship: 'I mean my husband now always says that if I said something and it's not what he wants me to say – oh your levels must be high'.

Reactions to insulin

The feelings and experiences associated with life on insulin therapy were complex and diverse and add some insight into the meaning that patients attach to the concept of quality of life. Both positive and negative feelings were identifiable.

Comments that on the surface appeared to be positive disguised more in-depth feelings. For example: 'Yes, I feel a lot better – the mood swings have gone, because before I suppose that it wasn't being in control and didn't know it', 'I accepted it but it never made no difference to me whatsoever' and 'it improved my life – I suppose – being on insulin'.

The negative comments outnumbered the positive ones and held some complex messages. For example: 'I got depressed – I don't know if it was the insulin', 'I felt down as well', 'I found it terrible – I wondered if my body was rejecting the insulin', 'I find that it really inhibits my lifestyle – I think that it's an effing nuisance' and 'I'm absolutely gutted because I never had hardly anything wrong with me in my life until I went on insulin'.

These findings reflected those that were identified within the literature review where an increase in depression was noted (Lustman *et al.*, 2000). It is difficult to identify a causal effect here other than to say that this is how the patients felt, irrespective of the physical factors. It would appear that on the basis of these collective comments the personal cost of insulin therapy for some is too high.

Patients came up with their own interpretations of what quality of life meant to them. For example: 'I'm still alive and doing what I want to do', 'living life to the full', 'Well, I want to be able to enjoy my kids' and 'I am just saying that I don't want to come to hospitals it's not a nice thing'.

Beliefs about insulin were associated with the amount prescribed and the association that was made with the severity of disease. For example: 'what do you take a day – bl**** h*** much lower than me', demonstrates a perception that the amount of insulin is important.

'Insulin doesn't make you put on weight, it alters the body so that your body is a lot better off than it was', 'I was told to take more insulin at night, but then it stores your fat at night times and that's when you put weight on'. These perceptions identify a gap in diabetes knowledge, and the reasons are twofold: either it is a sad reflection of the education process; or the patient has learnt from a peer or someone with whom they can relate more easily than the health care professional. The implication of this is that there needs to be a more thorough assessment of the patient's basic knowledge before an attempt is made to embark on the insulin-conversion process.

Losing control

When describing what life on insulin therapy felt like, the majority had negative feelings. This was for a number of reasons associated with power and control. Illustrative comments were 'since I have been put on insulin it has put me down further' and 'you have ruined me – I don't feel that it is my ideal ticket'. Some of this was fuelled by false expectations and disappointment, described as 'we were told this new person would emerge'. The underlying message here appears to be that the respondents felt they had been coerced by the health care professional to convert to insulin and therefore they felt that they had no choice. Consequently, they did not appear to have 'ownership' of their diabetes.

The minority who felt 'better' on insulin did so mainly as a result of a decrease in symptoms associated with poor glycaemic control. One respondent explained 'it is the best thing that ever happened to me – I find that my diabetes is virtually completely controlled'.

In addition, some used the 'sick' role to their advantage, that is, as a tool for ensuring that they got their own way. This correlates with the concept of control, except that in this situation the patient exerts control over other people. For example: 'I tell everyone and it's amazing how many people want to know' and 'if I go anywhere and I want quick service I say that I'm diabetic and they are all there [to give way]'.

Some respondents said that they were not sure whether insulin had made a difference to them. For example, 'it never made any difference to me' and 'I haven't felt any better'. In general, the majority of patients reported minimal or lack of personal benefit as a result of commencing insulin therapy. The meaning of quality of life to them was multifaceted and not necessarily related to their perceived negative or positive health status. This concurs with work undertaken by Snoek (2000), who felt that physical health does not appear to be a predictor of well-being or reported happiness.

Finally, the relationships that they formed with the health care professional and their experiences of the diabetes service as a whole had some impact on how they felt equipped to cope with life on insulin. Often, professionals were perceived to be unhelpful: 'Even with professional help there is no real support' and 'I don't think that I had enough education'.

Conclusion and recommendations

The underlying messages behind the findings are power and control, that is, the perceived power that patients feel the health care professional has over them and the subsequent loss of control that they experience as a consequence.

There is a range and diversity of interpretations of what is meant by power. It is usually described in two main forms: authority and coercion. When power is exercised and accepted as being legitimate, then it is regarded as authority. However, when it is not accepted as being legitimate, then it is perceived as coercion (Wilkinson and Meirs, 1999). This has been further expanded by

Table 2.2 Recommendations.

Recommendation 1	Glycaemic control is important; however, treatment goals should extend beyond this to incorporate the patient's personal goals.
Recommendation 2	More attention should be made to pre-assessment of the patient's perception of illness and health beliefs.
	Previous knowledge of diabetes needs to be assessed more thoroughly pre-conversion to dispel myths and misconceptions where possible.
	More in-depth exploration of the patient's fears and expectations before the conversion process is recommended (some patients may require more 'one-to-one' consultations with the diabetic specialist nurse)

Weber as 'the chance of a man or a number of men to realise their own will in a communal action, even against the resistance of others who are participating in the action' (Haralambos, 1985). The concept of empowerment is embedded in the current paradigm for effective diabetes management (Department of Health, 2001) in which the patient is encouraged to take responsibility for his or her own health management. The intention is that this enhances the patient's sense of control over his or her destiny.

The majority of respondents in this study had not come to terms with their diabetes. Few had managed to integrate insulin into their lives in a positive manner. Whether this was as a result of poor education, poor two-way communication, or both, is difficult to ascertain. In addition, there did not appear to be any identifiable differences between age ranges or gender. Nonetheless, the themes of power and control suggest that the manner in which health care information is delivered must be framed from the patient's perspective. If patients feel coerced or that they are not in control of their own destiny, they are less likely to adopt self-caring strategies that may limit future development of diabetes-related complications. The findings of this study, therefore, support the argument for patient empowerment. Table 2.2 highlights recommendations for practice.

Impact on practice

Changes have been made to the researcher's area of practice by altering the style, time span and content of the education programmes. This now includes weight management and enabling patients to take control of their diabetes earlier on in the insulin-conversion process. Patients are taught how to adjust their insulin, and to meet lifestyle needs within the first month following conversion to insulin. Most importantly, there is greater investment in developing partnerships with our patients that both support the empowerment model and readdress the balance of power in the patients' favour.

Part 3
Common partnership themes
Kimmy Eldridge

Introduction

Both papers are based on small but original research studies that were driven by the genuine desire to understand specific health issues from the patient's perspective. They are excellent examples of partnership working between professionals and patients. Treadwell aimed to find out what type of support and which measures help to sustain cessation of smoking. Young's study was carried out to find out whether conversion to insulin is always the best option for the patient.

The researchers claim that the main drive for both the studies was to seek to understand specific issues from the perspective of patients. They conclude that successful intervention is based on partnership that incorporates individual needs and goals. This section will examine the consistency with which partnership principles are applied in practice.

The research design and recommendations

In deciding the research aims, the researchers openly acknowledged the gap in their knowledge. This honesty engenders trust, a critical ingredient in partnership working (Lowndes *et al.*, 1997; Wildridge *et al.*, 2004). Their exploratory research design, which focuses on the experience of patients, promotes the notion that patients bring equal value to the partnership between researcher and participants. Thus, both papers suggest an interdependent relationship between the nurse researcher and the patient. This stance differs from the traditional paternalistic expert model of care, where the nurse is a professional, an expert, and the patient, in the sick role, is a receiver of expert care (MacGregor, 1998; Charles *et al.*, 1999; Steinhart, 2002). Within the scope of a small-scale project undertaken as part of master's degree studies, it is not possible to incorporate user involvement in the research design.

The thematic analysis is further testimony of the nurse researchers' willingness to spend time listening to the views and feelings of patients as research participants. The relationship that develops between the researcher and the participants is crucial if a genuine understanding of the problems faced by smokers and individuals receiving insulin therapy is to be achieved. This approach acknowledges patients as individuals in their own right, and as the main source of knowledge of their own experience (Gubrium *et al.*, 2002).

By contrast, in quantitative research design the researcher is detached and distanced from the participants (Spencer 1983). The participants are considered merely as sources of data (Carr 1994) and, in experimental research design, participants of the control and experiment groups are unaware of the true nature of the intervention because it is not possible, within the research design, to inform them if they have been assigned to the control or the experiment group (Cormack 1991).

Notwithstanding the strengths and weakness of quantitative and qualitative research designs, the justification of Treadwell's and Young's research and the study design reflects two of the six key principles of partnership developed by the Nuffield Institute for Health (for full principles please refer to Chapter 1):

- The acknowledgement of the need for partnership
- The development and maintenance of trust (Hardy *et al.*, 2000).

However, further scrutiny of the language used in the studies suggests minor inconsistencies in the translation of the partnership ideal into practice. Treadwell's first recommendation was that health care workers need to accept that relapse to smoking is a chronic condition and as such need to provide support for patients. This statement implies that relapse as a chronic condition is primarily the concern of the health care workers who need to adopt a proactive stance to provide 'support'; the role of the patient and his or her decision has not been made clear. This recommendation is inconsistent with the tone throughout the report and the remaining recommendations that reflect the principles of concordance.

Young's recommendations state the importance of incorporating the patient's personal goals into treatment aims. By acknowledging that the patient has personal goals, Young implies that the patient is goal-directed, thus shifting the patient from a passive to an active role in care. This pro-partnership stance is further supported by the suggestion that patients' perceptions of health and illness and knowledge of diabetes should be assessed as the basis on which to dispel patients' misconception of diabetes. The willingness to share knowledge with patients is indicative of shared control and partnership building (Henderson 2003; Wildridge *et al.*, 2004). However, the recommendations did not go far enough to reflect the principles of concordance – that patients should be offered choices in treatment.

Neither paper acknowledges the potential contribution of the 'expert patient' in the education and training of health care staff. Involving patients as service users in education has been promoted by the Department of Health (1994) and the NHS Executive (1996). It is not always practicable to involve users in curriculum development and there is a risk that user involvement is mere tokenism. Nonetheless, user involvement in education brings about a number of benefits; including helping to ground practice in reality, challenging existing approaches and providing a focus on partnership between professionals and users (Khoo *et al.*, 2004).

Shared aim and purpose

In Treadwell's study the shared aim of the patient and the nurse is to prevent relapse in cessation of smoking. In Young's study the nurse and the patients shared the same concerns: the effects of insulin therapy. This reflects the basic premise of partnership – the existence of a shared aim (Rummery, 2003; Wildridge *et al.*, 2004). In theory, it is this shared aim that draws the patient and nurse together, with both moving towards the achievement of the same vision (McLaughlin, 2004). However, both the diabetes and smoking studies found that partnership working remains a challenge to some health care staff.

These studies assume that both parties, the patient and the professional, want the same thing, i.e. for the patient to stop smoking and for the blood sugar to be controlled. In reality, there were underlying differences between what the patients wanted and the aims of the professionals. For example, in Treadwell's study, John had stopped smoking but wanted support so that he could continue so to do. The practice nurse suggested that he should delay until a more appropriate time (see below). Bill, in his effort to give up cigarettes, wanted a defined process with one appointment following another. The practice nurse asked him to phone up to make the next appointment, suggesting that the practice wanted a more flexible arrangement.

In Young's study, the participants wanted to feel well and live a life without restriction. The professionals wanted to achieve optimum glycaemic control. Given the differences, it seems inevitable that there will be tension and conflict between the patient and the professional. Conflicts in the professional–patient dynamics are recognised by policy makers and commentators (Wildridge *et al.*, 2004). The web site of a Cabinet Office project, which aims to assist voluntary and public sector organisations to work in partnership, identified 'managing inevitable conflict between partners' as one of the five stages in the lifecycle of a partnership (Cabinet Office, 2006). Feedback and emotional intelligence are two of the many measures proffered on the website as a means of working through the conflict.

It would appear that the health care professionals were unaware of the conflict in either study. This indicates that the relationship between the professional and the patient has not reached the first stage of the partnership life cycle as identified by the Cabinet Office's project: that is, connecting how the potential partners get to know each other and plan together.

Trust, understanding and support

In the smoking study, John had given up smoking for three weeks with the aid of nicotine patches that he had bought over the counter. Before Christmas he went to see the practice nurse for a prescription of these patches in order to continue to stop smoking. The nurse told him that Christmas and New Year are the wrong time to give up smoking and therefore he should not try to stop. She ignored John's view and imposed her assessment of the situation on him. Such an approach reflects the traditional model of care, where the nurse, as the expert, possesses knowledge and knows what is best for the patient. By contrast, the patient-centred care model advocated by the Royal College of General Practitioners highlights the importance of following the patient's cues, exploring the patient's own belief about the illness (in John's case, his readiness to stop smoking), and provides choice in treatment options (Campion *et al.*, 2002).

Patients with experiences similar to John's led the Pharmaceutical Society to introduce the concept of concordance in 1997 (Marinker, 1997) and the Government to introduce the expert patient initiative in 1999 (Department of Health, 1999b). If the nurses that John encountered had applied the principles underpinning these initiatives they would have listened to John and discussed with him when and how he should take nicotine patches to sustain his effort to stop smoking. Instead the nurse asked him for proof of his intention to stop smoking before prescribing nicotine patches. The behaviour of the nurse suggests that she did not understand John. Being understood is a basic human need. Demonstrating understanding through empathy is fundamental to helping relationship in nursing (Reynold *et al.*, 2000). John's experience of the nurse supports the findings of research that found that health care professionals show a low level of empathy (Reynold *et al.*, 2000). In Treadwell's study, such a failure in nursing led to an adverse patient outcome: John was angry. When the second nurse phoned to see how he was doing, he perceived it as yet another pressure. Unable to cope, he turned to smoking for comfort.

The need to feel understood is a theme that is shared by the participants in Young's study. One of the male participants talked about the argument he had had with his wife and her having a 'dig' about his insulin injections and the inflexibility of the evening meal-time. Another female participant felt that her husband made her blood sugar level the scapegoat when they had a disagreement. This attitude led the participants to feel unsupported and that they 'should not be ill at all'.

Support came in different forms for different individuals. John, who wanted to stop smoking, needed encouragement and non-judgemental attitudes from health care staff in order to motivate and energise him to take control of his craving for cigarettes. Others found the 'stop smoking' peer support group helpful. The importance of emotional support has been demonstrated by research evaluating disease-specific support groups (Zeigler *et al.*, 2003; Steginga *et al.*, 2004).

Emotional support is based on trust, which is a critical success factor in partnership working (Wildridge *et al.*, 2004) and the foundation of the nurse–patient relationship. Summer (2001) describes patients' vulnerability during 'illness-induced' interactions with health care staff and their yearning for the 'considerateness' of others. 'Illness' creates a need to trust and for help in coping (Miller, 1992). This demonstration of respect and trust includes self-awareness and communication skills. Communication skills are not an optional extra: John's nurse showed that without communication skills her knowledge and expertise were wasted and, as such, did not benefit John.

Power and empowerment

The behaviour of the nurse who told John his timing to stop smoking was wrong and who wanted proof that he was going to use the nicotine patches is evidence of the dominance of professional power over patients, and that nurses use persuasion to ensure that patients conform to nurses' understanding of 'appropriate' behaviour (Hewison, 1995). When health care professionals 'had a go at' or embarrassed the patient, e.g. John in front of his daughter, the patient felt belittled and disempowered.

In both studies, professionals exercised control over patients in many ways. Patients in Young's work reported that 'doctors don't tell you nothing' and that they wanted professionals to 'just be up front about it [information]'. Transferring knowledge and skills to patients to increase their competence, confidence and control is the hallmark of patient-centred care and requires a particular professional attitude and specific behaviours (Kennedy *et al.*, 2005).

Empowerment does not mean that patients must constantly make decisions about their own care. John found information about the nicotine patches helpful in his effort to stop smoking. Bill said he did as he was told, e.g. if it [what he should do] was written down on a piece of paper, he would be able to do it [stop smoking]. From both John's and Bill's perspectives, the information enabled them to exercise control over their situations. The nurse as the information giver is thus enhancing the patient's resources, which is the essence of partnership and empowerment (Rodwell, 1996; Freeth, 2001). By contrast, the participants of Young's study articulated their discontent when they felt they were not given a choice in the treatment of their condition. The lack of ownership of the treatment decision led one patient to continue to question 'why am I taking it [insulin]?'

Most participants in this study had not come to terms with their diabetes and had not integrated insulin into their lives in a positive manner. Unless the key prerequisites for concordance – power sharing, decision making, open discussion of all options, understanding the beliefs and perceptions of the patients (Marinker and Shaw 2003) – are achieved, education programmes alone (as part of the insulin-conversion therapy) will not improve ownership of treatment decisions. Lack of concordance will therefore persist.

Ultimately, the decision to stop smoking and maintain safe blood sugar levels while on insulin therapy rests with the patients. The participants in Treadwell's study acknowledged that 'it is completely down to me, it's me that's got to do it'. Such an attitude suggests that the individual is prepared to take responsibility and exercise control over his or her smoking behaviour, knowledge gained through experience, such as the effect of high blood sugar, enables adjustment and control.

Conclusion

These two studies reveal the complexity of partnership working with patients. Treadwell and Young show humanity and sensitivity to patients' needs in their research approach and seek answers to issues that concern patients. Their research design demonstrates genuine desire to work in partnership with their patients, and yet they were unable to translate this intention into consistent practice.

The research findings reveal that, in the main, doctors and nurses have retained their traditional, paternalistic approach to patient care. At best, they are not consistently giving information and sharing control in decision making. At worst, patients are humiliated and disempowered.

Patients in Young's study wanted to be involved in their care: they wanted information and have demonstrated that, through the experience of living with their diabetes and insulin, they have learnt about hyperglycaemia: 'I noticed with high blood sugars that I am really aggressive'. This particular patient is therefore more knowledgeable about his needs than health care professionals.

References

Bandura, A. (1977) Self-efficacy: towards a unifying theory of behaviour change. *Psychology*, **54**, 846–52.

Bernard, H. R. (2000) *Social Research Methods: Qualitative and Quantitative Approaches*. Sage Publications, London.

Borland, R., Segan, C., Livingston, P. and Owen, N. (2001) The effectiveness of callback counselling for smoking cessation: a randomised trial. *Addiction*, **96**, 881–9.

Bottorff, J., Johnson, J., Irwin, L. and Ratner, P. (2000) Narratives of smoking relapse: the stories of postpartum women. *Research in Nursing and Health*, **23**, 126–34.

Bradley, C. (2001) Importance of differentiating health status from quality of life. *Lancet*, **357**, 7–8.

Bradley, C. and Speight, J. (2002) Patient perceptions of diabetes and diabetes therapy: assessing quality of life. *Diabetes Research Review*, **18**(Suppl. 3), S64–9.

Brandon, T. H., Lazev, A. B. and Juliano, L. M. (1998) Very delayed smoking relapse warrants research attention. *Psychological Reports*, **83**(1), 72–4.

Brandon, T. H., Bradley, N., Juliano, I. M., Amy, B. and Lazev, A. B. (2000) Preventing relapse among former smokers: a comparison of minimal interventions through telephone and mail. *Journal of Consulting and Clinical Psychology*, **68**(1), 103–13.

Butler, C. C., Pill, R. and Scott, N. C. H. (1998) Qualitative study of patients' perceptions of doctors' advice to quit smoking: implications for opportunistic health promotion. *British Medical Journal*, **316**, 1878–83.

Cabinet Office (2006) *Partnership Guidance*. Cabinet Office, National Council for Voluntary Organisations, London (http://www.ourpartnership.org.uk/anncmnt/; last accessed 23 February 2006).

Callum, C. (1998) *The UK Smoking Epidemic: Deaths in 1995*. Health Education Authority, London.

Campion, P., Foulkes, J., Neighbour, R. and Tate, P. (2002) Patient centredness in the MRCGP video examination: analysis of large cohort. *British Medical Journal*, **325**, 691–2.

Carr, L. T. (1994) The strengths and weaknesses of quantitative and qualitative research: what method for nursing? *Journal of Advanced Nursing*, **20**, 716–21.

Charles, C., Whelan, T. and Gafni, A. (1999) What do we mean by partnership in making decisions about treatment. *British Medical Journal*, **319**, 780–2.

Ciechanowski, P., Hirsch, I. I. and Katon, W. (2002) Interpersonal predictors of HbA1c in patients with Type 1 diabetes. *Diabetes Care*, **25**(4), 731–6.

Cormack, D. (ed.) (1991) *The Research Process in Nursing*, 2nd edn. Blackwell Scientific, Oxford.

Curry, S. and McBride, C. (1994) Relapse prevention for smoking cessation. *Annual Review of Public Health*, **15**, 345–66.

Curry, S., Wagner, E. and Grothaus, L. (1990) Intrinsic and extrinsic motivation for smoking cessation. *Journal of Consulting and Clinical Psychology*, **58**(3), 310–16.

De Grauw, W., van de Lisdonk, E., van Gerwen, W., van den Hoogen, H. and van Weel, C. (2001) Insulin therapy in poorly controlled Type II diabetic patients: does it affect quality of life? *British Journal of General Practitioners*, **51**(468), 527–32.

Department of Health (1994) *Nurse, Midwife and Health Visitor Education: A Statement of Strategic Intent*. HMSO, London.

Department of Health (1999a) *Smoking Kills: A White Paper on Tobacco*. The Stationery Office, London.

Department of Health (1999b) *Our Healthier Nation – Saving Lives*. The Stationery Office, London.

Department of Health (2001) *National Service Framework for Diabetes: Standards Document*. Department of Health, London.

Department of Health (2003) *Statistical Bulletin 2003/21 Statistics on Smoking: England 2003*. Department of Health, London.

Douek, I. and Gale, E. (2001) The problem of weight gain on insulin treatment. In: *Insulin Made Easy* (ed. A. Barnett). Medical Education Partnership, London.

Freeth, D. (2001) Sustaining inter-professional collaboration. *Journal of Inter-Professional Care*, **15**(1), 37–46.

Furlow, L., O'Quinn, J. and Winslow, E. (1996) Research for practice. When the nurse says 'stop' smokers listen. *American Journal of Nursing*, **96**(3), 57.

Galvin, K. T. (1992) A critical review of the health belief model in relation to cigarette smoking behaviour. *Journal of Clinical Nursing*, **1**, 13–18.

Garcia, M., Schmitz, J. and Doerfler, L. (1990) A fine-grained analysis of the role of self-efficacy in self-initiated attempts to quit smoking. *Journal of Consulting and Clinical Psychology*, **58**(3), 317–22.

Gould, D., Pearce, C. and James, T. (2000) The role of the practice nurse in smoking cessation. *Clinical Effectiveness in Nursing*, **4**, 142–62.

Gubrium, J. and Holstein, J. (eds.) (2002) *Handbook of Interview Research – Context and Method*. Sage, London,

Haaga, D., Gillis, M. and McDermut, W. (1993) Lay beliefs about the causes and consequences of smoking-cessation maintenance. *International Journal of Addictions*, **28**(4), 369–75.

Hajek, P., Stead, L. F., West, R., Jarvis, M. and Lancaster T. (2005) Relapse prevention interventions for smoking cessation (Cochrane Review). *The Cochrane Database for Systemic Review*, Issue 2, 2005. Chichester, UK; http://www.cochrane.org/.

Harackiewicz, J., Sansone, C., Blair, W., Epstein, J. and Manderlink, G. (1987) Attributional process in behaviour change and maintenance: smoking cessation and continued abstinence. *Journal of Consulting and Clinical Psychology*, **55**(3), 372–8.

Haralambos, M. (1985) *Sociology, Themes and Perspectives*, 2nd edn. Bell & Hyman, Bungay, Suffolk.

Hardy, B., Hudson, B. and Waddington, E. (2000) *What Makes a Good Partnership? A Partnership Assessment Tool*. Leeds: Nuffield Institute for Health

Helman, C. (2000) *Culture, Health and Illness*, 4th edn. Butterworth-Heinemann, Oxford.

Henderson, S. (2003) Power balance between nurses and patients: a potential inhibitor of partnership in care. *Journal of Clinical Nursing*, **12**, 501–8.

Hewison, A. (1995) Nurses' power in interactions with patients. *Journal of Advanced Nursing*, **21**, 75–82.

Holloway, I. and Wheeler, S. (2002) *Qualitative Research in Nursing*, 2nd edn. Blackwell Science, Oxford.

Jarvis. M. (2002) *Patterns of Smoking Cessation and Relapse, and Evidence for the Efficacy of Relapse-Prevention Intervention*. Department of Epidemiology and Public Health, University College, London.

Kennedy, A., Gask, L. and Rogers, A. (2005) Training professionals to engage with and promote self-management. *Health Education Research*, **20**(5), 567–78.

Khoo, R., McVicar, A. and Brandon, D. (2004) Service user involvement in postgraduate mental health education. Does it benefit practice? *Journal of Mental Health*, **13**(5), 481–92.

Koopmanschap, M. (2002) Coping with Type II diabetes: the patient's perspective. *Diabetologia*, **45**(7), S18–S22.

Krall, A. E., Garvey, A. J. and Garcia R. I. (2002) Smoking relapse after 2 years of abstinence: findings from the VA Normative Aging Study. *Nicotine and Tobacco Research*, **4**(1), 95–100.

Lennox, A., Bain, N., Taylor, R., McKie, L., Donnan, P. and Groves, J. (1998) Stages of change training for opportunistic smoking intervention by the primary health care team. Part 1: randomised controlled trial of the effect of training on patient smoking outcomes and health professional behaviour as recalled by patients. *Health Education Journal*, **57**, 140–9.

Leventhal, H. and Cleary, P. (1980) The smoking problem: a review of the research and theory in behavioural risk modification. *Psychological Bulletin*, **88**, 370–405.

Lowndes, V., Nanton, P., McCabe, C. and Skelcher, C. (1997) Networks, partnerships and urban regeneration. *Local Economy*, **11**(4), 333–42.

Lustman, P. J., Anderson, R. J., Freedland, K. E., de Groot, M., Carney, R. M. and Clouse, R. E. (2000) Depression and poor glycaemic control: a meta-analytic review of the literature. *Diabetes Care*, **23**(7), 934–42.

MacGregor, S. (1998) From paternalism to partnership. *British Medical Journal*, **317**, 221.

Marinker, M. and Shaw, J. (2003) Not to be taken as directed. *British Medical Journal*, **326**, 348–9.

McLaughlin, H. (2004) Partnership: panacea or pretence? *Journal of Inter-Professional Care*, **18**(2), 103–13.

Marinker, M., Blenkinsopp, A. and Bond, C. (1997) *From Compliance to Concordance: Achieving Shared Goals in Medicine Taking.* Royal Pharmaceutical Society of Great Britain, London.

Miller, J. F. (1992) *Coping with Chronic Illness*, 2nd edn. F. A. Davis, Philadelphia.

NHS Executive (1996) *Education and Training Planning Guidance EL (96) 46.* NHS Executive, Leeds.

National Institute for Clinical Excellence (2002) *Guidance on the Use of Nicotine Replacement Therapy (NRT) and Bupropion for Smoking Cessation.* National Institute for Clinical Excellence, London.

Niaura, R., Abrams, D. B., Shadel, W. G., Rohsenow, D. J., Monti, P. M. and Sirota, A. D. (1999) Cue exposure treatment for smoking relapse prevention: a controlled clinical trial. *Addiction*, **95**(5), 685–95.

Niaura, R. and Abrams, D. B. (2002) Smoking cessation: progress, priorities, prospectus. *Journal of Consulting and Clinical Psychology*, **70**(3), 494–509.

Ogden, J. (2000) *Health Psychology: A Textbook.* Open University Press, Buckingham.

Pouwer, F., Snoek, F., Henk, M., Van der Ploeg, P., Ader, H., and Heine, R. (2001) Monitoring psychological well-being in out-patients with diabetes. *Diabetes Care*, **24**, 1929–35.

Prochaska, J. and DiClemente, C. (1983) Stages of processes of self-change of smoking: towards an integrative model of change. *Journal of Consulting and Clinical Psychology*, **51**, 390–5.

Reynolds, W. J. and Scott, B. (2000) Do nurses and other professional helpers normally display much empathy? *Journal of Advanced Nursing*, **31**(1), 226–34.

Ritchie, J. and Lewis, J. (2003) *Qualitative Research Methods: A Guide for Social Science Students and Researchers*. Sage, London.

Rodwell, C. M. (1996) An analysis of the concept of empowerment. *Journal of Advanced Nursing*, **23**(2), 305–13.

Rollnick, S., Mason, P. and Butler, C. (2000) *Health Behaviour Change: A Guide for Practitioners*. Churchill Livingstone, London.

Rose, M., Fliege, H., Hildebrandt, M., Schirop, T. and Klapp, B. (2002) The network of psychological variables in patients with diabetes and their importance for quality of life and metabolic control. *Diabetes Care*, **25**, 35–42.

Royal College of Physicians (2000) *Nicotine Addiction in Britain*. Royal College of Physicians, London.

Rummery, K. (2003) Progress towards partnership? The development of relations between primary care organisations and social services concerning older people services in the UK. *Social Policy and Society*, **3**(1), 33–42.

Schachter, S. (1982) Recidivism and self-cure of smoking and obesity. *American Psychologist*, **37**, 436–44.

Scotts, A., DiClemente, C., Carbonari, J. and Mullen, P. (1996) Pregnancy smoking cessation: a case of mistaken identity. *Addictive Behaviours*, **21**, 459–71.

Snoek, F. (2000) Quality of life: a closer look at measuring patients' well-being. *Diabetes Spectrum*, **13**, 24–35.

Speight, J. (2002) Assessing the impact of diabetes screening on quality of life or quality of health. *Diabetes Care*, **25**, 1893–4.

Spencer, J. (1983) Research with human touch. *Nursing Times*, **29**(12), 24–7.

Stapleton, J. (1998) Cigarette smoking, prevalence, cessation and relapse. *Statistical Methods in Medical Research*, **7**(2), 187–203.

Stapleton, J. (2001) *Cost effectiveness of NHS Smoking Cessation Services*. Action on Smoking and Health, London.

Steginga, S. K., Pinnock, C., Gardner, M., Gardiner, R. A. and Dunn, J. (2005) Evaluating peer support for prostate cancer: the prostate cancer peer support inventory. *BJU International*, **95**, 46–50.

Steinhart, B. (2002) Patient autonomy: evolution of doctor–patient relationship. *Haemophilia*, **8**, 441–6.

Sumner, J. (2001) Caring in nursing: a different interpretation. *Journal of Advanced Nursing*, **35**(6), 926–32.

Sutherland, G. (2003) Smoking: can we really make a difference? *Heart*, **89**(Suppl ll), ii25–ii27.

Testa, M. and Simonson, D. (1998) Health economic benefits and quality of life during improved glycaemia control in patients with Type II diabetes mellitus. *Journal of the American Medical Association*, **284**(17), 1490–6.

United Kingdom Prospective Diabetes Study (1998a) United Kingdom Prospective Diabetes Study 33 Group – Intensive blood glucose control with sulphonyureas or insulin compared with conventional treatment and risk of complications in patients with Type II diabetes. *Lancet*, **352**, 837–53.

United Kingdom Prospective Diabetes Study (1998b) United Kingdom Prospective Diabetes Study 38 Group – Tight blood pressure control and risk of macrovascular and microvascular complications in Type II diabetes. *British Medical Journal*, **317**, 703–13.

Urso, P. (2003) Match the best smoking cessation intervention to your patient. *American Journal of Primary Health Care*, **28**(1) Supplement: The 2003 Sourcebook for Advanced Practice Nurses, pp. 12–21.

Varni, J. W., Burwinkle, T. M., Jacobs, J. R., Gottschalk, M., Kaufman, F. and Jones, K. L. (2003) The PedsQL in Type I and Type II diabetes: reliability and validity of the pediatric quality of life inventory generic core scales and Type I diabetes module. *Diabetes Care*, **26**(3), 631–7.

Walling, A. (2002) Type 2 diabetes quality of life and early insulin therapy. *American Family Physician*, **65**(4), 529–750.

West, R., McNeill, A. and Raw, M. (1998) Smoking cessation guidelines for health care professionals. A guide to effective smoking cessation interventions for the health care system. *Thorax*, **53** (Suppl 5 Pt1), S1–18.

West, R., McNeill, A. and Raw, M. (2000) Smoking cessation guidelines for health care professionals: an update. *Thorax*, **55**, 987–99.

West, R., McNeill, A. and Raw, M. (2003a) *Meeting Department of Health Smoking Cessation Targets. Recommendations for Primary Care Trusts.* NHS Health Development Agency, London.

West, R., McNeill, A. and Raw, M. (2003b) *Meeting Department of Health Smoking Cessation Targets. Recommendations for Service Providers.* NHS Health Development Agency, London.

Wildridge, V., Childs, S., Cawthra, L. and Madge, B. (2004) How to create successful partnerships – a review of the literature. *Health Information and Libraries Journal*, **21**, 3–19.

Wilkinson, G. and Meirs, M. (1999) *Power and Nursing Practice.* Macmillan, London.

Williams, G. and Pickup, J. (1999) *Handbook of Diabetes*, 2nd edn. Blackwell Science, London.

Wiltshire, S., Bancroft, A., Parry, O. and Amos, A. (2003) 'I came back here and started smoking again': perceptions and experiences of quitting among disadvantaged smokers. *Health Education Research*, **18**(3), 292–303.

Zeigler, L., Smith, P. A. and Fawcett, J. (2004) Breast cancer: evaluation of the common journey breast cancer support group. *Journal of Clinical Nursing*, **13**, 467–78.

Zinman, B. (1997) Translating the Diabetes Control and Complications Trial (DCCT) into clinical practice; overcoming the barriers. *Diabetologia*, **40**, S88–90.

CHAPTER 3

Mental health

Introduction

Peter J. Martin

This chapter varies from the format of the rest in this book. Firstly, the same author, Nick Wrycraft has written both papers. Secondly, the papers represent two forms of scholarly activity not included elsewhere in this book. The former paper examines an aspect of mental health care with reference to relevant literature and the latter reports on an evaluation of an educational programme. The editorial decision to include the papers was based upon the focus within each paper on partnership working within mental health services.

The author is a mental health nurse who has held a number of posts within the local health sector. Currently, Wrycraft works for a Higher Education Institution (HEI), but at the time of writing he had a dual role working in research and development and preparing Primary Care Graduate Mental Health workers in an HEI.

The first paper was prepared as a submission for part of an MSc scheme during which students undertook an elective placement. In the paper Wrycraft describes and analyses an unnamed assertive outreach service in which he was placed. The paper integrates theory and practice through discussion about issues raised within the placement. Indicators concerning how partnerships with service users function within such teams are examined.

The second paper was prepared by Wrycraft as a commissioned report to the National Institute for Mental Health in England whilst employed in research and development. This paper is an extract from the commissioned work, an evaluation of the 'Trail Blazers' course. The course brings together small groups of primary and secondary care providers. The groups design and deliver small-scale multi-agency mental heath projects that improve local service provision and facilitate joint working, leadership, and integrated working. The section of the report included in this book draws out specific areas of the evaluation that relate to partnership between different mental health service providers.

Part I
Assertive outreach
Nick Wrycraft

Intention

This chapter examines:

- The theoretical background to assertive outreach services
- Practice within assertive outreach teams
- Key practice issues in establishing partnership with service users

Introduction

This paper reflects on partnership working with service users in an assertive outreach team. Two different forms of knowledge inform the paper: practical experience through placement and theoretical research in the form of an extended literature review. To facilitate understanding on the part of the reader and presentation on the part of the writer, practical experience is described in the first person.

The practical experience described consisted of a two-day placement spent with an assertive outreach team, the operational policy for which derives from a single model of assertive outreach. The model is examined from the perspective of partnership-based intervention with service users. Assertive outreach is considered at a macro political level before considering how it is applied at the micro level of service delivery. Comparison is drawn between the assertive outreach service and my own Trust.

Background

I elected to undertake a study of assertive teams in order to facilitate improvements in the service in which I was based. At the time of writing I was employed in an adult mental health service. In this service there were a number of service users with complex or long-standing needs who periodically required in-patient admission.

I had noted that service users were often discharged back into deleterious social or environmental circumstances, exposing them to repeated failure within the community and the prospect of further episodes of in-patient admission (Hannigan and Cutcliffe, 2002). Hemming *et al.* (1999) identify that regular service users were frequently admitted to in-patient services for social rather than specific health reasons. This problem occurred in my locality, so I wanted to visit another area to learn how they provided a service to this particular client group.

Assertive outreach aims to reduce hospital admissions and improve service users' quality of life. This is achieved through a 'time-unlimited' team model that seeks to engage service users' in their own home environment (Sainsbury Centre for Mental Health, 1998). Appropriately targeted assertive outreach can provide a method of averting crises (Hemming *et al.*, 1999). In doing so, it substantially reduces the cost of hospital care whilst improving health outcomes and satisfaction through engaging service users as partners in their care (Hannigan and Cutcliffe, 2002).

Assertive outreach is perceived by the UK Department of Health as an integral component of the developing network of mental health services in the UK. The expressed intention was to create 260 assertive outreach teams nationwide by 2003, 360 crisis resolution teams and 50 early intervention in psychosis teams, which will represent a flexible, responsive, community-based network of mental health services (Department of Health, 2000a). Yet while, internationally, assertive outreach has substantial research-based support, there has been a more mixed and sceptical response in the UK (Burns and Priebe, 2004; Ford and King, 2005; Tyrer and Simmonds, 2003; Sainsbury Centre for Mental Health, 2003).

There are several different models of assertive outreach currently in existence, ranging from the Strengths Model to the Rehabilitation-Oriented Model to Clinical Case Management and Assertive Community Treatment (Ryan, 1999). This paper considers Stein and Test's ACT Model (1980), though this is not necessarily the model of choice for all outreach UK teams. The choice of assertive outreach model should be based on assessment of the type and extent of local need and available resources (Sainsbury Centre for Mental Health, 2001). The team, which is the subject of this paper, is a 'Beacon Site of Good Practice' (Department of Health, 2000b, p. 26). It has been described as having a '… structured programme of dissemination, where practitioners can visit and take away evidence to help shape their own services' (Dodd, 2000).

Literature review

Assertive outreach was developed in the USA approximately 30 years ago (Dodd, 2000). Studies in the USA indicate that assertive outreach has been successful in avoiding relapses and hospital admissions (Ramon, 1996. p. 124). These findings are supported within Onyett and Smith's (1999) discussion of the strengths of assertive outreach. Onyett and Smith (1999, p. 70) note that assertive outreach helps with the management of 'difficult to engage' clients and that users and carers expressed a preference for this form of care above others. Furthermore, recent reviews of international literature suggest additional benefits, including improvements in the clinical status of users, independent living, better social functioning, improved quality of life and increased compliance with medication (Onyett and Smith, 1999, p. 70).

The Department of Health reported that, of 23 controlled studies with assertive outreach, 61% reported significant reductions in hospital admissions (Department of Health, 1999, p. 47). Hemming *et al.* (1999) cite research suggesting a 35% reduction in hospital admissions and an increase in the number of days that service users spent in stable accommodation. Further work cited by Hemming *et al.* (1999) identified fewer admissions requiring police involvement, fewer compulsory admissions and less use of crisis services, evidently due to the higher frequency of contact and earlier detection of relapse which assertive outreach can provide. However, the UK700 Group (1999) found evidence suggesting that assertive outreach teams did not produce better results than conventional community treatment teams (see also Thornicroft and Goldberg, 1998).

While there is a significant body of international research supporting the efficacy of assertive outreach, consideration needs to be given to the specific cultural and environmental requirements particular to the UK. Such factors may influence both the design of assertive outreach team services and potential outcomes (Onyett and Smith, 1999, p. 70; Hemming *et al.*, 1999).

Fidelity to the model is necessary to establish effective assertive outreach teams (Dodd, 2001) and deviation may result in reduced value and impact of the assertive outreach approach (Meaden *et al.*, 2004). The failure of recent research to demonstrate the same benefits found from earlier assertive outreach teams has been attributed to the lack of fidelity to a single model (Sainsbury Centre for Mental Health, 2001). While Hemming *et al.* (1999) contend that fidelity to the model is important, they only advocate this to the extent of embodying the central characteristics of the model; however, they do not do not specify which of these features they prioritise.

Strict adherence to a specific model may not be the only reason for the limited impact of assertive outreach in some areas of the UK. The failure of research in the UK to demonstrate the positive effects of experience elsewhere may be due to several factors. Community mental health teams already work effectively in many of the areas where assertive outreach would demonstrate change, and other factors such as culture, bureaucracy and resources should be considered (Ford and King, 2005).

Case study

I will now examine the practical application of the model of care employed by the assertive outreach team and describe how partnership was developed. The team adhere to Stein and Test's (1980) model of Assertive Community Treatment (ACT), which is defined as (Department of Health, 1999):

> ... a clinically effective approach to managing the care of severely mentally ill people in the community. Staff providing comprehensive assertive outreach care for clients will visit them at home, act as an advocate, and liaise with other services such as the GP or social services. Help is usually needed to find housing, secure an adequate income, and sustain basic daily living – shopping, cooking, and washing for example.

The following case study is a short narrative account of an experience whilst on placement.

Case study – Steve

The service user, a young single man 'Steve' (a pseudonym), lived with his aunt. I visited Steve with a member of the assertive outreach team who was known to, and knew, Steve well. On arrival we discussed with Steve what he would like to do and he chose to go for a drive in the countryside. On the journey Steve pointed out local sites for my benefit and bought some lunch at a fast food restaurant. We then returned to his home, where the team member had a brief talk with Steve's aunt about his mental health. Steve's manner was friendly and he did not express concern that his mental health was being assessed during our visit; he talked openly and comfortably with the team member and I felt they had a good rapport with each other.

Due to the informality of the intervention and the social nature of the activities carried out I doubted whether Steve felt as though he was receiving care, yet he appeared to value the contact. The team member explained that his goals were to motivate Steve, orientate him to the local community and facilities and support Steve's aunt while monitoring his mental health. This appeared to achieve an amicable 'trade-off', despite Steve and the team apparently having differing perceptions of the contact.

Practice in assertive outreach teams

Assertive outreach aims to: '... improve (service users) material and social environment and train in activities of daily living, social relations and work' (Onyett and Smith, 1999, p. 70). The assertive outreach team's philosophy aims to maintain clients in the community, as opposed to preparing them for community life. This is an important distinction and demonstrates that assertive outreach is not a pedagogical enterprise. While some service users may engage in training or employment, others may not. Including training and employment goals within a definition of assertive outreach is flawed, because it introduces unrealistic expectations of the service and might undermine its ability to engage service users.

Service comparison

Box 3.1 compares my own area of practice and that of the team where I was on placement. The area I visited was geographically disparate; it was largely rural but contained several large towns. In contrast, my locality is a relatively small town in a contained area within a coastal peninsula. Consequently, less time is lost waiting in traffic or travelling long distances on visits (Dodd, 2001). The length of in-patient stay in the area I visited was often calculated in terms of years. In my locality in-patient bed stays are generally much shorter. The staff reported that there was no access to rehabilitation or respite beds within the community. In my locality there are a number of residential rehabilitation beds available.

Effective functioning of assertive outreach teams requires a range of available services within the network to provide choice for service users (Hemming

Box 3.1 Comparison of services

Placement service	Comparator	Local service
■ Large area including rural and large urban areas	■ Geographical location ■ Length of in-patient stay	■ Contained rural area with small town ■ Significantly shorter
■ Long term, often measured in years	■ Residential rehabilitation facilities	■ Available in the local community
■ Not available in the local community	■ Inter-agency working	■ Well developed and long-standing inter-agency working
■ Limited inter-agency working		

et al., 1999). Such services are enhanced by good links with the independent and voluntary sector (Sainsbury Centre for Mental Health, 2001). In my locality there is a proactive and well-developed local voluntary and independent sector for service users and an active relationship with the statutory mental health services. Despite the absence of a formally constituted assertive outreach service locally, there are already the elements of assertive outreach. For example, within our day services there is a member of staff who goes to the gym with clients and takes them to snooker halls. The efficiency with which assertive outreach is organised and implemented determines the quality of service provided at the point of delivery (Ryan, 1999). But this invokes the question of whether services need to be developed that adhere to the strict criteria of assertive outreach or whether a more adaptable model would be more acceptable which might evolve out of the current service.

Interventions

The help offered by an assertive outreach service may involve, '... shopping, medication, sorting out benefits, money matters and home visits' (Ramon, 1996, p. 124). I observed that the therapeutic outcome of the interventions actively engaged service users in a productive and stable relationship with the team. A member of the team explained that he advised clients on welfare benefits as a method of creating trust, as people would more readily feel a rapport with someone who secured them tangible gains. However, pragmatic interventions of this kind need to be supported by sound therapeutic rationales and justified using appropriate assessment tools that are frequently evaluated.

Interventions should also benefit the service user's mental health and be framed in a nursing context in order to have a professionally credible basis. The risk of not grounding the work is that assertive outreach is regarded as a treatment that attempts to engage 'at any cost'. This may ultimately erode the ethical basis supporting the treatment and the health care professional may feel their role to be diminished in value (Onyett and Smith, 1999). Furthermore, service users may become suspicious of services goals, believing help offered is a bribe to secure engagement (Smith, 2001). While assertive outreach is perceived as engaging on a social level with clients and removing boundaries, surprisingly the team were acutely aware of their boundaries.

Referrals

Referrals are assessed by a detailed review of the service user's previous history of contact with the mental health services, focusing on why they had not engaged successfully. Two members of the team, generally from different disciplinary and professional backgrounds carried out assessment (for example a psychologist and nurse or occupational therapist and nurse). Particular consideration was paid to the service user's interests and personality and how they might be appropriately engaged based on this information. Assertive outreach should function within the context of mental health services, acting as an overall network and adding to the network of service choices for users (Hemming *et al.*, 1999). Such an integrated service is more likely to assist users to find a service that provides them with individualised care and equips health care professionals with extra treatment options; particularly when existing service provision for these clients is clearly failing (Ryan, 1999).

In order to create a 'seamless service' each team member had a detailed knowledge of all the service users with whom the team were working. Each person had a named worker on the team with whom they worked most frequently. This team member had the speciality or skills that most matched the service user's needs. However, the team managed their visits from the staff available at the time. The rationale was to prevent named workers being left 'owning' problems, or people returning from absences to confront a backlog of visits. These measures demonstrate the practical application of supportive team working in an acute need setting and were consistent with the team's own written evaluation of its strengths.

Support and assertive outreach teams

The emotional health of practitioners in assertive outreach teams exerts a direct influence on relationships with service users and clinical outcomes. It is therefore important to provide support for the team and accentuate the importance of good emotional health. In a comparison between job satisfaction, burnout and work experiences of assertive outreach teams and community mental health teams (CMHTs) there were higher ratings for emotional exhaustion in assertive outreach teams than CMHTs, and significant differences in some burnout components between teams using different models (Billings *et al.*, 2003). Another study identified the quality of client–therapist interaction as a factor contributing to reducing admissions and length of admission under assertive outreach (Meaden *et al.*, 2004). Practitioners and teams who are supported will be better situated to develop effective partnerships with service users. Features such as teamwork, supervision, leadership, effective management, a clearly developed strategy, vision, a plan for implementing the change and how it will be integrated within the existing network of services are crucial areas of emphasis which ought to be considered in planning assertive outreach and pivotal to its success (Onyett and Smith, 1999).

The nature of the work of assertive outreach teams exposes team members to a high level of stress and responsibility. Working as Care Programme Approach (CPA) Care Coordinators on a long-term basis for people with acute and ongoing mental health problems involves assuming a high level of responsibility and accountability for the care of service users, who by definition are in a high-risk group. Unsurprisingly there is anecdotal evidence of difficulty in recruiting team members.

In order to maximise the potential for support within the team in which I was placed there were twice-daily meetings to discuss caseloads, share information and provide peer support. The team described an atmosphere similar to many community mental health teams where colleagues provided informal support, helped by the regular meetings as a means of ensuring that the team had intimate knowledge of all the service users with whom the team were involved. Details of visits and therapeutic input were also shared between the team regardless of the named care coordinator, and clinical supervision was recommended as good practice and a central component of the team functioning. In other assertive outreach teams all of the team members, including those of other non-nursing disciplines and those without a professional qualification, were encouraged to seek clinical supervision at least once a month in addition to receiving regular line management supervision (NEST, 2005).

Staffing issues

The creation of a specialist multi-disciplinary team may be regarded as expensive, but available research on assertive outreach suggests it is a cost-effective treatment (Onyett and Smith, 1999). This may be measured in relation to savings occurring in in-patient bed occupancy (in terms of both duration and volume of service users). It may also be cost-effective because non-qualified support workers can undertake much of the work after the assessment stage (Ramon, 1996. p. 124).

The team employed a mix of qualified and non-qualified support staff, which was reported to be effective within the team's working procedures. Support workers in assertive outreach teams need a health or social care background as well as life experience (Dodd, 2001). In addition to good team support and clinical supervision they need to have the personal and professional resources to deal with the potential challenges of community work in the absence of a professional qualification.

Service users and employment

Community-based assertive outreach offers the potential for targeted therapeutic activity in the community, an example being employment. Fewer people with enduring mental illness are in employment compared with those with a general disability; this is an area where improvement could be made with those service users who have the ability and potential to enter employment (Sayce, 2000). No relationship has been found between psychiatric diagnosis and work skills, although symptoms were found to be more severe in the unemployed (Anthony *et al.*, 1995). I feel this provides an indicator of the possible benefits that assertive outreach could offer towards facilitating greater social inclusion for service users within the community.

Accessing employment and occupational opportunities is essential for service users, even where they have acute and ongoing mental health problems. The ageing population has created the necessity for more adults of working age to be in employment and has encouraged government-led innovations (for example Job Centre Plus) to facilitate employment opportunities for all sectors of society and an increasing emphasis on social inclusion among vulnerable and minority groups (Office of the Deputy Prime Minister, 2004).

Conflicting views

Those working in assertive outreach risk becoming trapped between conflicting demands. The public, through the media, appear to demand that teams are instruments of coercion by which mental illness is managed in society. Conversely, user groups perceive the role as curtailing the civil liberties of service users in the community (Hannigan and Cutcliffe, 2002; Ryan, 1999). The conflicting views may balance this polemical and emotive debate. The ethos of partnership which underpins the teams may be maintained and assertive approaches become neither too coercive, yet proactive enough to reach the hardest to engage clients.

Due to the acute and ongoing nature of the mental health problems of those service users with whom assertive outreach teams become involved, the team with which I was placed concentrated on working with service users by understanding them in the context of their lives. This contrasts with conventional therapeutic-led models that work to reinstate mental health and impose normality on service users. A consequence of this approach is that there is an acceptance that mental ill health will continue to be a part of service users' ongoing lives, and the service is vulnerable to the criticism of lowering the goals of treatment. However, I believe that assertive outreach represents a growth in realistic expectations of what mental health services can offer. Yet it is important that these services continue, proactively, to strive to offer creative solutions for their clients with access to as full a range of opportunities as possible, including occupation and employment. Clinical and management support, together with good team relationships and a genuine interdisciplinary approach, will ensure that the service can provide useful and practical assistance for service users with acute ongoing mental health problems to function within society.

Conclusion

This paper has reported on observed practice within an assertive outreach team, with consideration of the relevant literature. Assertive outreach can add an extra dimension to the range of existing services available. Central to its effectiveness is the flexibility and ability of the staff in interpreting and implementing the spirit of assertive outreach into practice. In my area I feel that the single most important consideration in the development of a service is to clarify the remit of an assertive outreach team. From various discussions I have had with other staff in my Trust it has often been assumed that assertive outreach can be regarded as early intervention treatment of clients who may become long-term service users and those already with multiple admissions who are hard to engage. It is necessary to identify one or other client group as eligible for referral to an assertive outreach team – embracing both extremes will only spread services too thinly.

Part 2
An evaluation of the 'Trail Blazers' course
Nick Wrycraft

Intention

This chapter examines:

- The background to the Trail Blazers course
- Delivering the Trail Blazers course
- Partnership issues emerging from the Trail Blazers course

Introduction

This paper reports on part of an evaluation of the multi-disciplinary education programme. The Trail Blazers course, which is the subject of this evaluation, was organised by National Institute for Mental Health in England (NIMHE) (now Care Services in Partnership – CSIP). The evaluation was an independent commissioned project by CSIP, carried out by the author.

Background

The Trail Blazers course was developed by Tylee, Armstrong and King (Brown *et al.*, 2002) and has been conducted at six sites across the UK. Participants are given the opportunity to develop skills in specific in areas through undertaking the Trail Blazers course. These skills include leadership, innovation and dissemination in relation to good practice in mental health care. Practitioners apply to the course as pairs, one of whom works in primary care and the other in secondary care. During the course the pairs decide on a project to jointly progress during the life of the course.

Key literature review

The majority of service users with mental health problems remain in primary care and are not referred to secondary services (Department of Health, 1999; Kendrick *et al.*, 1994; National Institute for Clinical Excellence, 2002; National Institute for Mental Health in England, 2004; Tunmore, 2002). Primary care providers therefore need to be equipped with the skills necessary for the effective management of mental illness. This objective was made explicit by the current UK Department of Health policy in documents such as the National Service Framework for Mental Health (NSF) (Department of Health, 1999).

To support primary care mental health the Government made a financial commitment and established the Workforce Action Team (WAT) in August 2001. The WAT was to ensure that the workforce was '... sufficient and skilled, well led and supported to deliver high quality mental health care' (Workforce Action Team, 2001a, p. 2). A separate report was prepared for primary care recommending that education and training be strengthened and developed (Workforce Action Team, 2001b). The Trail Blazers course promotes the integration of services and access to skills and expertise at the primary and secondary care interface.

Brown *et al.* (2003) was the only study evaluating Trail Blazers; it examines the first cohort of the West Midlands scheme in 2002. The evaluation was qualitative, with data sources including application forms, module evaluations, the researcher's experience as a participant observer of the modules and interviews with 13 of the 14 participants on the course. The evaluation demonstrated short-term effectiveness in terms of participant reaction, knowledge and changes in professional practice. Further research was recommended including a longitudinal study.

The Trail Blazers course, supported by National Institute for Mental Health in England Eastern, brings together leaders from primary and secondary care settings in a forum that supports innovation and the development of good practice. The course has no set curriculum and adopts an 'action learning' approach (Brown *et al.*, 2003).

The study

The study evaluated the experience of participants and facilitators on the Trail Blazers course in relation to the identified aims and objectives for the course. This paper examines some of the findings of that evaluation.

The qualitative study used several data sources, including application forms, module evaluations and semi-structured interviews with participants and facilitators. Informants were drawn from a single Trail Blazers cohort and included participants (24) and facilitators (4). Triangulation of the different data sources strengthened the design of the study.

Brown *et al.*'s (2002) Trail Blazers evaluation adopted Kirkpatrick's (1967) hierarchy as a framework to structure the evaluation. Brown *et al.* (2002) identified several limitations in the use of this framework, notably that the Trail Blazers course produced a number of 'intangible outcomes' (Brown *et al.*, 2002). To build on the lessons of the previous evaluation, this project adopted a flexible frame of reference. Themes taken from application forms, module evaluations and interviews were integrated into subsequent interviews, and cross-referenced with other data.

Findings and discussion

Professional background

The course comprised ten pairs or groups; eight were pairs and two were groups of three participants. During the course one pair withdrew after the first module

Box 3.2 Participants by professional background

Group	Designation	Designation	Designation	Designation
1	Community Mental Health Team Manager	General Practitioner (special interest)		
2	Community Psychiatric Nurse (Modules 1 and 2)	Senior Occupational Therapist	Occupational Therapist (Module 3)	
3	Counsellor	Team manager		
4	Service Improvement Manager	Service Director (Modules 1 and 2)	Research Facilitator	
	Service Improvement Manager (Module 3)			
5	Clinical Improvement Manager	General Practitioner		
6	Joint Commissioning Manager	Specialist Health Visitor		
7	Carer/Trainer	Project Manager	Project Manager	
8	Ordained Minister of Religion	Ordained Minister of Religion		
9	General Practitioner	Community Psychiatric Nurse		
10	Community Psychiatric Nurse	Practice nurse		

NB
- The course consisted of 'groups' and 'pairs'; for ease, both will be referred to as 'groups'.
- The 'ideal' model described by Brown et al. (2002) consisted of pairs comprising primary and secondary care representation.
- Variance was avoided where possible, but became necessary because of the range of initial applications and subsequent commitments.
- Some participants were unable to attend all modules, and substitutions were made, as indicated, with the agreement of the groups by the facilitators.
- Groups were multi-professional except for Group 8 and Group 1 (module 3 only).

due to a lack of support from their employing organisation. Box 3.2 identifies the pairs/groups who participated during the three modules by profession.

A case study from a Trail Blazers participant

The following is a narrative account of attending the Trail Blazers course from an independent counsellor participant.

> My expectations were not all specific. I was aware of a gap in our local mental health services and the idea of creating a service to fill in this gap, but I felt stuck, without a clear way forward and a lack of management insight and support. I was looking for some enthusiasm and I felt that Trail Blazers could offer me some direction. Although our project was vague I thought this was not a problem and that Trail Blazers would allow for this.
>
> Working in pairs was stimulating and the space given to us was such a treat. We realised how difficult it had been to find quality time to work in partnership in our work environment. We were able to focus on how to move forward with our ideas. It was a relaxed space and yet very productive.
>
> One part of our project (early intervention) was very much within the original expectation, although it is now clearer and more evolved. The other part (relating to improving services within our Social Centre) did take shape at Trail Blazers beyond our original expectations. We had ideas about what could be done and we were able to stretch out those ideas during the work as a pair that we had not been able to do elsewhere. The knowledge/insights and confidence gained on the course certainly exceeded my expectations.
>
> The style of facilitation was suitable to meet my needs. Facilitation was fluid, open and caring. I think we were made to feel comfortable and open to the experience. I felt the balance between time with our project partner and facilitated sessions was good. I was surprised at how able I had been to sustain concentration and focus throughout the day and that the variety had kept me going and interested. The icebreakers were all memorable. They brought some humour that drew me in the group and dissipated any anxiety.
>
> The first self-awareness session (getting to know ourselves) reminded me that the project was not only about practical issues and how I could set the service up, but also what skills or personal attribute did require developing or strengthening to increase my chances of success. This group exercise was meaningful to me because I could identify within the group a role model with the specific attributes or skills required and be inspired. The 'critical friend' groups also served to enrich our ideas. No other course provides a choice of sessions on topics we choose. That was great, the session on commissioning was strategically important to our project.

Interviews

The author undertook seven semi-structured interviews. Data included is from four interviews with facilitators and three with participants (*n* = 3); two facilitators and two participants were interviewed as pairs. The following reports some of the evaluation findings that add dimension to partnership between service providers.

1   The Trail Blazers course had no set curriculum; it was designed to be developmental and to be shaped by the needs of the participants. Three modules of two days duration included (1) reflection on learning needs and plans; (2) facilitated sessions and participant feedback; (3) facilitated sessions, feedback and peer review by group/facilitators.

    Participants noted that projects in which the groups engaged did not progress consistently throughout the course. Some projects moved smoothly through to completion whilst others encountered problems that had to be resolved before they could progress further. As a result the course was not linear, but a series of loops. Participants felt that this replicated the real world in which they worked, and the review sessions allowed groups to develop problem-solving skills from the experiences of others.

    One facilitated session that was particularly well received by participants was 'critical friends'. These sessions were a form of peer supervision where participants presented their ideas, progress, resources and plans to the rest of the group for critical appraisal. The participants stated several times in the evaluation forms that the 'critical friends' process and the way that it was used to elicit non-judgemental constructive criticism and sharing of ideas and information was extremely useful in the developing the projects.

    The working partnerships that developed in the groups mimicked the experiences of participants in their workplaces. One facilitator reported that the first module enabled participants to establish ways of working with others and the course team. Relationships were established on a flexible basis, with each partner making a distinct contribution. Flexibility was important because it allowed the projects to progress at a rate that was manageable for the individual participants. The relationships were subject to both internal and external forces. The groups had to (internally) establish ways of working which were acceptable to the members, which required discussion and negotiation of the power differentials that existed within the groups. Externally, the groups were engaged in projects that required the involvement of others from the workplace. Groups spent time deliberating the most effective way of communicating and sharing the innovation with colleagues.

2   The course attempted to balance project-dedicated time and facilitated time. A carer participant stated 'it was a chance to get away from the phone and

emails to concentrate on the project'. From the module evaluations, participants felt that an appropriate balance was attained between project and facilitated time. Facilitators experienced greater anxiety about balancing time as they felt a responsibility to facilitate the groups and sessions, whilst participants expressed that they preferred to be self-directed. Another facilitator gave the example of extending project time during a module; partners working late into the evening; and some working on presentations early the next morning.

The course was 'light on content' a facilitator noted, but the greatest benefit came from the development of working relationships between partners. One of the facilitators felt that, in planning the next cohort, the course ought to adopt a more definite structure in order to be able to map the process more clearly.

Balancing facilitated and project time within the course is comparable to identifying time for innovative work within busy work schedules. Participants therefore valued this 'thinking space'. Unfortunately, protected time dedicated to engaging in original thinking about such projects is perceived as a luxury within the workplace.

3 Participants were drawn from a wide range of mental health work, both statutory and non-statutory. Data from interviews and evaluations indicate that the range of participant backgrounds positively enhanced the learning experience. Participants and facilitators felt that the cohort group provided a pool of support, expertise and human resource to supplement the partnerships. The evaluation sought to ascertain whether those from a non-NHS background felt that the course had been of use to them and whether they had been able to learn and contribute. A carer who attended the course was paired with two project managers employed by the NHS. Her feedback was positive, feeling that it 'showed partnerships in care... carers should be tapped into for their own experience'.

Linking up participants into partnerships enabled projects to be progressed more effectively, but also motivated members through a shared sense of purpose. Participants and facilitators felt that that, where groups pre-existed there had been an opportunity to build upon the relationship. This was perceived as an advantage over those who were paired together either by the course organisers or sent on the course by their employer.

The course enabled people to work together, integrating different components of a project into a single cohesive whole. In order to do this project teams had to define the shared goals and aspirations in a very explicit fashion. By 'preparing the ground' at the outset projects moved forward from a sound foundation shared by all.

4 The projects on which participants worked during the Trail Blazers course were not required to have any particular form. The course has no assessment or expectation of output. Whilst groups are encouraged to work on a single

project several groups modified their project during the course. An ordained minister of religion stated that the course had assisted his group to 'to bring our project into focus and make it realistic and workable'. Initially he had been concerned that the course would be health orientated and 'we would be out of our depth', but he had been pleased by how the course had met his learning needs.

The following are statements from application forms that illustrate the aspirations and aims of the participants on commencing the course. These have been selected to represent the range of projects on the course.

I would like to be involved in a programme aiming to improve the delivery of mental health. Still and often I hear dissatisfaction from service users about the care they receive further adding to their current distress. I know we could and should do better. I aspire to establishing a mental health service that better meet(s) the needs of its users. (*Independent Service Manager*)

To prepare a strategy for the PCT and risk assessment in reviewing the National Service Framework for Mental Health, i.e. review policies (and) protocols already in place and measure the PCT against standards and targets. To improve performance and develop awareness both in the local and wider health economy so as to improve working practices for the benefits of patients. (*Joint Commissioning Manager*)

The selected projects for this course have been grouped and presented in Boxes 3.3–3.6. Nine projects are listed; the omission is because one group with-

---

Box 3.3 Projects 1: An intervention or clinic

For example:

- A memory clinic
- An educational initiative targeted at residential home/in-patient nursing staff working with older people with dementia
- A clinic to assist with the physical health care needs of those with an acute mental health problem in the community
- A mental health triage service receiving referrals from general practice
- An independent telephone helpline service for carers of people with mental health problems

Box 3.4 Projects 2: A policy or strategy

- A mental health strategy for a PCT
- A mapping exercise as a prelude to a mental health strategy for a PCT

Box 3.5 Projects 3: A funding proposal

- A proposal to change the role of spare premises at an existing independent mental health service in the community

Box 3.6 Projects 4: Raising awareness

- An incentive to raise awareness of the mental health needs among the religious community

drew. Facilitators noted that, in general, outline projects were too large and needed to be scaled down to make them manageable within the framework of the course. However, one pair came onto the course with the intention to develop a mental health strategy for a Primary Care Trust; as this was their goal there had been no suggestion that this ought to be revised and the project was completed.

Participants in the Eastern region and West Midlands courses varied in the projects they selected to work upon. The West Midlands projects were primarily educational and consultation exercises (Brown *et al.*, 2002). In contrast, two of the Eastern region projects were educationally orientated and one concerned preparing a bid to remodel its service. The other six projects were on improving the efficiency with which mental health services in primary care were organised and delivered.

On completion of the course all of the projects had shown significant progress:

- The mental health triage service was operational and had assessed 26 referrals.
- The telephone helpline was due to be launched.

- The memory clinic was being launched and had been subject of a published article in the National Institute for Mental Health in England publication *Eastforwards*.
- A mental health strategy for a PCT was completed during the course.
- The mental health awareness initiative was functioning and was now supported by a leaflet, with development of a video in progress.
- All of the other projects made progress during the course.

The broad range of projects developed by the groups demonstrates the appeal of the Trail Blazers course. Groups were able to work on a variety of issues whilst engaging in a shared learning experience. In order to complete the projects, groups engaged in partnership, working with others with whom they may not normally engage. A measure of success of the course is the completion of projects and the concomitant demonstrable improvement to the scope and quality of local mental health services.

Recommendations

This partial report on the Trail Blazers course highlights a number of issues pertaining to effective partnership working.

- Effective partnerships should involve all stakeholders, for example statutory and non-statutory providers, service users and carers.
- Employing organisations supported and were committed to the projects that were most successful.
- Participants valued both facilitated and dedicated sessions. However, in order to work and think creatively participants needed dedicated 'thinking time' within the course where they could develop the projects.

Conclusion

This report is an educational evaluation rather than a systematic research study. The design of the evaluation was concerned with capturing the essence of the Trail Blazers course rather than attempting the form of evaluation carried out by Brown *et al.* (2002) using a recognised model of educational evaluation.

Part 3
Common partnership themes
Peter J. Martin

Introduction

The two papers included in this section provide some useful insights into the development of partnership working. Paper one examines how an assertive outreach team works in partnerships with service users. Paper two focuses on partnerships between primary and secondary care mental health services.

As was noted in the introduction to this section, these papers are not presented as original research. The contribution of these papers is primarily in strengthening the research-based papers that comprise the other chapters. The papers present views of partnership from different perspectives, but an analysis of the work indicates that there are a number of common themes running throughout them. That comparison can be drawn between the two papers suggests that the skills underpinning partnership working are transferable. Thus skills can be used as effectively within a therapeutic encounter with a service user as in project working with service providers.

Multi-professional and multi-agency

Professional groups are guided by a distinct view of the world and apply different knowledge and skills to the framing and solving of problems. A distinct facet of both of Wrycraft's papers is collaborative work between different agencies and professions. The strength of this approach is to enable a problem or issue to be examined from a range of perspectives.

The assertive outreach team attended by Wrycraft undertook multi-professional assessment of service users and ensured follow-up by different members of the team. This is supported by Smith and Morris (2003) who recognise that each team members will make a unique contribution to the support of the service user.

The Trail Blazers course encouraged multi-agency groups to focus on the delivery of single projects. Bringing the focus of a multi-professional and multi-agency group to bear on a problem enabled groups to share strategies and resolve problems more effectively. Adams (2005, p. 36) suggests that the current drive for inter-professional education is a defence against the loss of unity and the recognition of difference that exists within modern societies. The Trail

Blazers course enabled different perspectives to be acknowledged by the group and, consequently, the problem to be understood from all angles.

Partnership working can be strengthened by the incorporation of different perspectives. This assumption may relate more to stakeholders than professional groups or agencies. The engagement of professionals and agencies in partnership working has value because of the perspective that they bring to a problem. However, it may be more valuable to engage them because they are stakeholders. As stakeholders they may be in a position to either facilitate or sabotage decisions and outcomes.

Outcomes

In the first paper, Wrycraft argues that effective partnerships require engagement between practitioners and service users. Similarly, in the second paper, project work was facilitated when every member of the group was engaged in the process. Engagement with the process is the consequence of individual investment in the process through the anticipated attainment of unique and tangible goals.

Wrycraft suggests that partnerships within assertive outreach teams are based on tangible goals. Service users engage with practitioners on the basis of goals that are perceived as beneficial. The practitioner and the service user may have different goals, but the encounter ensures that both attain their desired outcomes. For example, in the case study that Wrycraft presents, Steve attains his desire to 'go for a drive in the countryside' and associated outcomes. At the same time the key worker is able to undertake an assessment of client and carer, Steve and his aunt.

In the Trail Blazers course the projects contain the outcomes. Primary and secondary mental health care workers may have goals that they wish to achieve through the project that may be different. However, attainment of the project outcome will enable both sets of goals to be attained. Hudson *et al.* (1997) indicate that a 'shared vision' between participants is a means to overcoming barriers to inter-agency collaboration. Within the definition of shared vision, Hudson *et al.* refer to specifying user-centred goals and the mechanism for achieving these goals.

For example, one of the projects concerned establishing a triage service for general practitioners. For general practitioners, the potential impact of such a service would be great. It would enable people with mental health problems to be seen more rapidly, create less anxiety for members of the practice and create opportunities for improved primary and secondary care working. For the secondary care services the triage system would improve the quality of referral and speed up access to service for those with greatest need. Hence the outcome of establishing the triage service will enable both primary and secondary care service partners to attain their goals, which can be specified in terms of outcomes for service users.

A professional basis for partnership

Assertive outreach based on engagement 'at all costs' was rejected in Wrycraft's first paper. He argued that engagement should be based upon a clear professional role within the service; however, this aspect of partnership in Wrycraft's papers is less tangible. It is not clear how a professional basis for partnership is established or how it operates.

Wrycraft appears to suggest that, where partnership exists between service user and nurse, the nurse should draw upon nursing as a professional basis for his or her practice. However, Wrycraft also argues that assertive outreach is, in itself, a coherent policy built upon research evidence. In order for assertive outreach to attain positive outcomes much is made within the literature about the importance of fidelity to the service model. Team members are required to possess a clear professional perspective in addition to demonstrating fidelity to a service model. A conflict of perspectives would appear to be inevitable at some point, particularly as one of the strengths of assertive outreach is the multi-professional constitution of the service.

A similar argument can be postulated in relation to multi-professional/agency working. Wrycraft argues coherently that the Trail Blazers course established partnerships between different professional groups and agencies. This multiple perspective was a strength in that projects were more complete and did not suffer from a blinkered, uni-professional, view. However, the context in which Trail Blazers was run was relatively neutral, with self-selected participants, established ground rules and facilitators. It is reasonable, therefore, to assume that those with professional backgrounds were open to working in a collaborative manner; and the carers, counsellors, ministers etc. were capable of coherently presenting the significance of their own role in health and social care. In this 'safe' context, outcomes would be achieved through shared ambition.

Health and social care is infused with power, which operates between the different service and professional interests. Adams argues that the 'credibility of inter-professional collaboration rests on its capacity to contain the ambiguity that arises between the different sources of its legitimacy, each source with its own separate competing interests, purposes and rationality' (Adams, 2005). In more traditional health and social care environments that do not specifically aim to be power-neutral, a strong professional perspective may distort multi-agency discussion in environments. Psychiatrists or service managers may be able to assert their authority over team decision making simply because they are perceived by others to be powerful. Therefore a strong professional perspective may be useful in partnership working, but only if the outcome reflects the perspective of all participants rather than simply the moist powerful voice.

Support

Support for people working in partnership is multi-faceted and a significant component of partnership working. Papers one and two appear to suggest that support people working in partnerships require internal and external space if they are to be effective.

Internal space can be described as 'thinking time' – time when people can pause and reflect upon their work. This can be attained either independently through the use of reflection upon practice or with assistance through supervision. Wrycraft identified that support for staff working in assertive outreach teams included various forms of supervision. Supervision in different guises is considered fundamental to contemporary practice, but is still not universally adopted by practitioners.

In the Trail Blazers course, participants valued the protected time they were given to develop projects; this can be regarded as internal space. During these times in the programme participants were given time and space to sit and explore with peers the progress of their projects. This has the elements of a supervisory relationship in that it incorporates support, education and focus of the task (Hawkins and Shohet, 1989).

External space is the support given by employers and organisations to the development of good practice. As a new service, created in response to Department of Health directives, it is apparent from Wrycraft's report that the assertive outreach team received support to develop the service at a strategic and operational level.

It is evident through examination of the titles that none of the projects undertaken by the Trail Blazers participants could be considered as 'rocket science'. The projects appear to be sound and sensible developments of practice. However, the space and time to think about designing, developing and delivering the project is often not available to people. Hence such projects often remain in people's heads and at an abstract level.

Effective partnership working requires support. Firstly, people need to be 'open' to the possibility of how partnership working might benefit themselves and others. Secondly, people need to be supported to engage with others in partnership. Where people do not have access to internal or external space in which to consider partnerships there is a tendency to return to isolationist working practices that do not benefit anyone.

Flexibility

Partnership working, as has been noted, involves people working collaboratively to some shared purpose. Health and social care is dynamic, with change being brought about through changing political, social and health trends. Consequently, partnerships need to be flexible in the short and long terms.

In assertive outreach, the team were required to offer services that were flexible, responsive and community-based. This might imply *ad hoc* working partnerships between service users and service providers' functions. The flexibility with which assertive outreach teams operate is flexibility whilst remaining focused on service goals. This permits services to be delivered on a highly individualised basis focused on meeting the needs of the individual.

It is possible to see flexibility underpinning partnerships developed within the Trail Blazers course. Groups worked together to develop projects, but during the life of the project there was a continuous process of review and renegotiation to ensure that participants were all engaged with the process. Without this process occurring group members would become disillusioned with the process and disengage.

Conclusion

The two papers by Wrycraft have highlighted a number of points found to be consistent in both service user and inter-agency focused partnership. These papers have demonstrated how working in partnership can create positive outcomes and service developments. The points that have emerged through analysis of Wrycraft's papers are interrelated and form the basis of good practice in partnership working.

References

Adams, A. (2005) Theorising Inter-professionalism. In: *The Theory–Practice Relationship in Inter-Professional Education*. Higher Education Academy, London.

Anthony, W., Rogers, E., Cohen, M. and Davies, P. (1995) Relationships between psychiatric symptomatology, work skills and future vocational performance. *Psychiatric Services*, **27**(2), 145–6.

Billings, J., Johnson, S., Bebbington, P., Greaves, A., Priebe, S., Muijen, M., Ryrie, I., Watt, J., White, I. and Wright, C. (2003) Assertive outreach teams in London: Staff experiences and perceptions. Pan-London assertive outreach study part 2. *British Journal of Psychiatry*, **183**, 139–47.

Burns, T. and Priebe, S. (2004) The survival of mental health services: a pressing agenda? *British Journal of Psychiatry*, **185**, 185–90.

Brown, C., Bullock, D. and Wakefield, S. (2002) *Evaluation of the 'Trail Blazers' Mental Health Teaching the Teachers Course in the West Midlands*. University of Birmingham, Birmingham.

Brown, C., Wakefield, S., Bullock, D. and Field, S. (2003) A qualitative evaluation of the 'Trail Blazers' teaching the teachers programme in mental health. *Learning in Health and Social Care*, **2**(2), 74.

Department of Health (1999) *National Service Framework for Mental Health*. HMSO, London.

Department of Health (2000a) *NHS Plan – A Plan for Investment, a Plan for Reform*. HMSO, London.

Department of Health (2000b) *NHS Beacon Learning Handbook: Spreading Good Practice Across the NHS*, Vol. 1. HMSO, London.

Dodd, T. (2000) Born in the USA. *Mental Health Practice*, **4**(1), 25–6.

Dodd, T. (2001) Clues about evidence for mental health care in community settings. *Mental Health Practice*, **4**(7), 10–14.

Ford, K. and King, M. (2005) A model for developing assertive outreach: meeting local needs. *Mental Health Practice*, **8**(10), 34–6.

Hannigan, B. and Cutcliffe, J. (2002) Challenging contemporary mental health policy: time to assuage coercion? *Journal of Advance Nursing*, **37**(5), 477–84.

Hawkins, P. and Shohet, R. (1989) *Supervision in the Helping Professions*. Open University Press, Buckingham.

Hemming, M., Morgan, S. and O'Halloran, P. (1999) Assertive outreach: implications for the development of the model in the United Kingdom. *Journal of Mental Health*, **8**(2), 141–7.

Hudson, B., Hardy, B., Henwood, M. and Wistow, G. (1997) *Interagency Collaboration: Final Report*. Leeds: Nuffield Institute.

Kirkpatrick, D. (1967) Evaluation of training. In: *Training and Development Handbook* (eds. R. Craig and L. Bittlel). McGraw-Hill, New York.

Meaden, A., Nithsdale, V., Rose, C., Smith, J. and Jones, C. (2004) Is engagement associated with outcome in assertive outreach? *Journal of Mental Health*, **13**(4), 415–24.

Kendrick, T., Burns, T., Freeling, P. and Sibbald, B. (1994) Provision of care to general practice patients with a disabling long term mental illness: a survey in 16 practices. *British Medical Journal*, **311**, 93–8.

National Institute for Mental Health in England (2004) *Enhanced Services Specification for Depression Under the New GP Contract*. National Primary Care Research & Development Centre and The University of York in partnership with the North West Development Centre of National Institute for Mental Health in England.

National Institute for Clinical Excellence (2002) *Depression: The Management of Depression in Primary and Secondary Care: Second Consultation*. National Institute for Clinical Excellence, London.

NEST (2005) The assertive outreach team – one year on. *Linking Hands*, **18**, 3–6.

Office of the Deputy Prime Minister (2004) *Mental Health and Social Exclusion: Social Exclusion Unit Report*. Office of the Deputy Prime Minister, London.

Onyett, S. and Smith, H. (1999) The structure and organisation of community mental health teams. In: *Serious Mental Health Problems in the Community: Policy, Practice and Research*, 2nd edn (eds. C. Brooker J. Repper), pp. 62–86. Baillière Tindall, London.

Ramon, S. (1996) *Mental Health in Europe: Ends, Beginnings and Rediscoveries*. Macmillan, London.

Ryan, P. (1999) *Assertive Outreach in Mental Health*. NT Books, London.

Sainsbury Centre for Mental Health (1998) *Keys to Engagement: Review of Care for People with Severe Mental Illness Who Are Hard to Engage with Services*. Sainsbury Centre for Mental Health, London.

Sainsbury Centre for Mental Health (2001) *Mental Health Topics: Assertive Outreach*. Sainsbury Centre for Mental Health, London.

Sainsbury Centre for Mental Health (2003) *Mental Health Topics: Assertive Outreach*. Sainsbury Centre for Mental Health, London.

Sayce, L. (2000) *From Psychiatric Patient to Citizen: Overcoming Discrimination and Social Exclusion*. Macmillan, Basingstoke.

Stein, L. and Test, M. (1980) Alternatives to mental hospital treatment: Conceptual model, treatment programme and clinical evaluation. *Archives of General Psychiatry*, **37**, 392–7.

Smith, I. (2001) Bladerunners. *Linking Hands*, **16**, 3–7.

Smith, M. and Morris, M. (2003) Assertive outreach. In: *Psychiatric and Mental Health Nursing* (ed. P. Barker), Ch. 45. Edward Arnold, London.

Thornicroft, G. and Goldberg, D. (1998) Has community care failed? *Maudsley Discussion Papers*, Numbers 1–10. Institute of Psychiatry, London.

Tunmore, R. (2002) Liaison mental health nursing in community and primary care settings. In: *Mental Health Liaison: a Handbook for Nurses and Health Professionals* (eds. S. Regel and D. Roberts), pp. 65–95. Bailière Tindall, Edinburgh.

Tyrer, P. and Simmonds, S. (2003) Treatment models for those with severe and comorbid personality disorder. *British Journal of Psychiatry* (Supplement), **44**, 15–18.

UK700 Group (1999) Comparison of intensive and standard case management for patients with psychosis: Rationale of the trial. *British Journal of Psychiatry*, **174**, 74–8.

Workforce Action Team (2001a) *Workforce Planning, Education and Training: Adult Mental Health Services: Executive Summary*. HMSO, London.

Workforce Action Team (2001b) *Workforce Planning, Education and Training: Adult Mental Health Services: Special Report*. HMSO, London.

CHAPTER 4

Information giving

Introduction

Peter J. Martin

This chapter comprises two papers and a critical review that extracts common themes relating to partnership working from two studies. Eastbrook and Reynolds are Patient Care Coordinators for General Medicine and Elderly Medicine respectively at a district general hospital. The papers report on two small-scale studies undertaken as part of a Masters degree.

The focus of the studies is on information giving, and the papers examine this process from different perspectives. Eastbrook's paper is concerned with the experience of nurses and patients, whilst Reynolds concentrates on the experience of carers. The papers assume that information-giving is part of the role of the nurse. From this start point the authors attempt to understand the processes by which information is disseminated and the factors that impact upon the dissemination. Eastbrook and Reynolds draw upon their extensive experience within the practice environment and the associated wealth of knowledge and skills they have accumulated.

Eastbrook and Reynolds sought and obtained approval to undertake the studies through the NHS Research Governance Framework and local Research Ethics Committee. The studies were undertaken under the supervision of the Department of Health and Human Sciences at the University of Essex.

The first paper highlights the importance of giving good quality, timely information to patients in order for them to take part in decision making and exercise choice in their care. The study demonstrates the need to provide patients with good quality information and resources about any diagnostic investigation that they may undergo whilst an in-patient in hospital.

The second paper examines the interaction of staff with carers and the significance and impact of this interaction on the patient's journey. The study looks at how carers seek information and their experience of this process and compares this with the nurses' perception of giving information.

Part I
Nurses' and patients' experience of giving and receiving information about diagnostic investigations
Sue Eastbrook

Intention

This chapter examines:

■ How nurses perceive their practice of giving information to patients
■ How patients experience receiving information
■ The gaps between patients' and nurses' perceptions of information giving and receiving
■ Ways of improving nursing practice by meeting patients' need for information

Introduction

This study sought to understand the perception of nurses and patients in relation to 'information giving and receiving' prior to diagnostic investigations. The findings from this study were used to develop a strategy for unmet needs and improve services within the local NHS Trust.

Background

The researcher is a Patient Care Coordinator for Medicine at a district general hospital. The role is pivotal in ensuring that patients have a pathway of care that is timely, informative and specific to their needs. The main area of responsibility is coordination of care for patients within the first 24 hours of admission, encouraging them to take an active role as partners in health care provision. Reflection on practice by the researcher led to the recognition that patients were not always given choice or involvement, especially after the initial period on the medical assessment unit. Once admitted to general wards it was particularly apparent that there was a lack of appropriate and timely information particularly about prospective diagnostic investigations. The researcher's concerns were substantiated by increased evidence that poorly informed individuals were less able to manage their health and treatment, have more anxiety and less favourable psychological outcomes (Caress, 2003; House and Stark, 2002; Kessels, 2003).

Key literature review

The researcher was only able to locate a small number of studies that investigated either content or context of information dissemination to patients prior to diagnostic investigations. Those studies that were located explored the outcomes of information giving and communication with relationship to patients undergoing surgical procedures (Hughes, 2002; Clements and Melby, 1998; Wallace, 1985; Mordiffi *et al.*, 2003; Mayberry and Mayberry, 2001). Previous studies were dated and did not investigate what the patient wanted to know or what nursing staff felt the patients should know before investigations were undertaken. The studies reviewed that were most relevant were researched in America, indicating that this is an area of health care that is under-developed in Britain.

Partnership in care between patients and health care professionals is recognised by governmental, regulatory and professional bodies as good practice. An increasingly informed and aware public expect to play an active role in decisions about their own care. However, patient participation requires health professionals to provide patients with timely and appropriate information. Nurses are often the practitioners who have the most contact with patients; therefore they are in an ideal position to ensure that specific information is given in a context that maximises the patients' understanding of the process.

The literature demonstrates that patients remain dissatisfied with the information that they receive from health care professionals. This includes poor delivery by health care professionals in relation to timing, quality and quantity of information (Audit Commission, 1993; NHS Executive, 1999; Mills and Sullivan, 1999; Coulter *et al.*, 1999; Cable *et al.*, 2003). Furthermore, professionals who cannot provide patients with consistent information cannot expect concordance or for patients to be reassured about pending interventions. Patients should not have to seek out information or pass uninformed through the Health Service (Nicklin, 2002).

The study

The primary aim of the study was to understand how nurses and patients perceived the current practice of information giving and receiving. A secondary aim was to explore the dynamic interactions between patients and nurses and to understand how this affected the information-seeking behaviour of patients.

A qualitative design was adopted for the study using one-to-one semi-structured interviews with patients and nursing staff.

Eight patients were interviewed. This group were being cared for on medical wards and had recently been the subject of diagnostic investigations. The patients were interviewed about their experiences of undergoing medical investigations with specific reference to the quantity and quality of the information received about the various tests.

Seven qualified nurses working on the same wards as the selected patients were also interviewed. The interview schedule was based around the issues raised by the patient group in relation to quality and quantity of information.

This method was considered appropriate as it gave respondents the opportunity to describe their experiences in their own words (Cormack, 1996). Decisions about study design were informed by literature reviewed during the project development. Thematic analysis was used to locate key themes within these data.

Findings and discussion

From the analysis of the data generated from the narratives by both patients and staff three themes emerged:

- Communication and knowledge
- Passive attitudes and trust
- Partnership of care

Communication and knowledge

The nurses' narratives suggested that communication was not recognised as an important aspect of patient care. Nurses reported that effective communication with patients was hampered because of time constraints and staffing levels in relation to the physical workload of the workplace. The primary focus of care was ensuring that the 'hands-on care' was completed before time could be allocated to talking to patients about their treatment.

If communication was considered a nursing intervention in its own right, the same importance would be placed on explaining aspects of treatment in a timely manner to patients as providing nursing care to meet hygiene needs. This would consequently reduce patients' anxiety and increase their knowledge of the treatment that they were to undergo (Price, 2004; Mayberry and Mayberry, 2001; Kennedy, 2001).

In order to communicate information, nurses must have the appropriate knowledge and resources. The narratives in the study suggest that respondents did not possess such knowledge and resources. Coulter *et al.* (1999) have already noted that such a lack of knowledge of treatment options and their effects by health care professionals is unsatisfactory. Nurses need to be motivated in order to create systems to allow the information to be given to patients in a usable format. The narratives from both groups of respondents did not reflect that nurses took ownership in information giving.

The nurses and patients interviewed stated that nurses did not know about investigations because they were not based on specialist wards where specialist knowledge about investigations was available and in common usage. This implies that nurses were not motivated to locate such information on behalf of patients for whom they were providing care. It would be unwise to simply chastise nurses for poor motivation, as the situation is complex, with a number of factors to be considered. Nurses' responsibilities have grown more varied and complex, with priorities centred on documentation and technology, leaving communication as a skill that nurses must foster in order to enhance patient care (Breisch, 1999). Furthermore, Cortis and Lacey (1995) link deficient information-giving to patients being admitted to wards that are not designed for certain medical conditions.

The study showed that the general quality of the information on wards about diagnostic investigations was perceived by respondents to be poor. The nurse respondents felt that it was an area of practice to which they had given little consideration. They expressed little awareness that patients needed good quality information at the time when they were informed that they needed to have a specific test. Studies have shown that poor quality information and information that is not given in a timely manner is of little benefit to patients (Cortis and Lacey, 1995; Coulter *et al.*, 1999; Arthur, 1995; McIntosh and Shaw, 2002; Kinrade, 2002).

Patients described feeling anxious about being subjected to a diagnostic test about which they had minimal information and for which they were consequently unprepared. Whilst some patients did comment that they had worried unnecessarily, this is hindsight and cannot be offset against the anxiety caused before the test. The gulf that existed between the nurses' perception and knowledge of the test and that of the patients was substantial; nurses expressed surprise that patients visualised investigations to be any different to reality. This finding was also reached by Wilson-Barnett (1990, p. 91), who stated that the most common fear expressed was fear of the unknown and that anticipation was often tainted by fantasies.

As a consequence of receiving deficient information, patients were placed in a dependent and disempowered position. Patients expressed that late or insufficient information resulted in an inability to prepare for and plan the day. Patients reported that they were unable to get information about how long they would be off the ward, or if they needed to stay in bed for any length of time. This is an example of the dissatisfaction that patients have when nurses do not give sufficient and timely information about their treatment (McColl *et al.*, 1996).

Patients did not want detailed or complex information about diagnostic tests or investigations. However, information considered useful included: whether it would be painful, how long it would last, and where it would take place. The information requested by the patients in this study already appears in the literature as pertinent questions that should be asked prior to investigations (Stevens and Dowd, 1999). This article, however, concluded that there had not been research, to date, that clarified the information content required by patients (Stevens and Dowd, 1999).

Information given by nurses varied significantly in terms of its quality. Good quality information was often associated with nurses who had previous experience of the relevant tests and could give a first-hand account of what the patient should expect. Experienced nurses in the participant group were able to give examples of patient information about investigations based on prior knowledge of clinical situations.

Nurse respondents reported that they assumed that patients knew more about investigations that they actually did. These assumptions were based on the quantity and depth of detail contained within television programmes and the media. This is supported by literature that recognises that today's patients are better educated and better informed about medical treatments and technologies (Stevens and Dowd, 1999; American Academy of Orthopaedic Surgeons, 1996; Jensen, 1987). This method of obtaining knowledge does not apply to all patients and assumptions about the patient's knowledge base should not influence information giving. Furthermore, patients should expect a relationship with a health care professional based on trust. This is very different from opportunistically encountering a diagnostic test on a television programme made for the purposes of entertaining/educating a mass audiences rather than informing the individual.

Nurses expressed that they did not consider all diagnostic procedures to be therapeutic interventions. Consequently, information about tests was only offered when expressly sought by patients. Examples of the patient's responses were discussed with the nurses during their interviews and they acknowledged that investigations were interventions and they should give information to patients prior to having them. Some nurses find changing practice very difficult (Pediani and Walsh, 1999), and historically nurses have not given this type of information to patients, as it was not considered a nursing task (le Tourneau, 2004).

Passive attitudes and trust

Nurses acknowledged that they did not always give information to patients prior to diagnostic tests. Some respondents accounted for this by arguing that patients took a passive role in relation to their health care. 'Patient' conjures up a vision of someone lying patiently in bed waiting for a medical doctor or nurse (Neuberger and Tallis, 1999). Respondents suggested that patients should sometimes take responsibility for asking questions; they should accept some responsibility in obtaining the information they needed. Duxbury (2000) argues that the 'passive patient' is a product of our health care system and such patients were once perceived as ideal patients. Nurses reported that elderly patients, a highly vulnerable and disempowered group, were the most passive. Whilst this group may retain an archaic perception of health care systems, nurses may unconsciously encourage this group to be passive by not disseminating information.

Although modern health care encourages the patient to be active in their care (Department of Health, 2001b), nurses do need to be proactive in ensuring that the right conditions are created in which a dialogue can take place. Despite this, Redwood (2002) suggests that the aim of health care appears to be to improve the knowledge base of health professionals rather than that of patients by giving them information. Nurses have a legal and ethical responsibility to ensure that information is delivered to patients in a format that they can understand about all aspects of their care (Greenwood, 2002).

Stratified sampling was not undertaken in relation to the age of the patient group. However, the findings indicated that the older age group were more accepting of a passive health culture. This is consistent with the findings of Woodward and Wallston (1987). In such a culture patients were discouraged from asking questions, and accepted treatment as directed by health care professionals. This type of culture is underpinned by non-verbal consent, known as implied consent, a term that is often abused by health professionals. An assumption is made that simply by coming into hospital, or by the nod or smile, the patient agrees to undergo any intervention, regardless of the level of information possessed by the patient. The literature reviewed also suggested that patients who were not given information were not able to contribute in their partnership of care (Greenwood, 2002).

Partnership of care

The study demonstrated that an equal partnership of care between patients and nurses did not exist. Where nurses had information about investigations, as a general rule, they did not share this knowledge with patients in their care. This model of health care is not patient-centred and cannot be seen as best practice. White (2002) states that all patients have the right to information, as their care is a partnership, not a one-way system with power held by health professionals.

Patients may choose not to know specific details, but this is the exercise of choice that can only be made if choice is offered at the outset. Nurses reported that they felt that some patients did not want to know information about investigations, because it might make them worry more about what the procedure involved. Such reasoning is patronising and incongruent in a contemporary health care system; it does not encourage patient empowerment or the patient's right to make an informed choice of treatment (Scott *et al.*, 2003; Cable *et al.*, 2003; Gert, 2002). The patient culture may exhibit passivity, but this culture is perpetuated by the dominant attitude amongst health care teams. Culture change for patients is peripheral to the continued perception of education by health care staff as being time-consuming and one-way traffic rather than a dialogue (Redwood, 2002).

Recommendations

Nurses need to recognise which patients adopt a passive role in their health care and why. This knowledge can be used to create an individualised strategy to address their learning needs. Patients need to be assisted to define their information needs and identify how best these needs might be met. Such assistance may come from nurses, but equally may be the role of advocacy and expert patient services.

A competency-based educational programme needs to be implemented at ward level. This would allow nurses to develop an awareness of the information needs of patients and how to formulate a baseline assessment. Staff should be given the opportunity to observe each investigation that patients on their wards may require. This will ensure that staff can communicate information based on first-hand knowledge in 'real life' situations.

The hospital's intranet service, 'patient line' system, and patient information resources should be updated and include information about investigations carried out in the hospital. These resources should be accessible to patients as well as staff. Link nurses should be nominated to liaise with departments that perform diagnostic investigations in order to ensure that updated information is available on the ward. In order to improve the knowledge that nurses have of diagnostic investigations it is recommended that a folder is made available on each ward containing literature about investigations that patients may undergo whilst in hospital. This can also be used as a teaching resource for nurses.

Ward Managers, Speciality Matrons and Clinical Skills Practitioners need to be made accountable for educating staff about the importance of communicating all aspects of care to patients. It is recommended that Ward Managers cascade the findings of this study to their staff at ward meetings in order to reassert the importance and professional responsibilities associated with good quality communication and information giving.

Implications

If these recommendations are not adopted, patients will not have an equal partnership in their care, and will continue to be misinformed and experience undue anxiety. By allowing current practice to continue nurses will be failing in their duty of care. By implementing the recommendations practice will be enhanced and patients will have an increasingly individualised approach to their learning needs and be better informed about impending diagnostic investigations.

Conclusion

The study has demonstrated the need to provide patients with good quality information and resources about any diagnostic investigation that they may undergo whilst an in-patient in hospital.

The central finding was the lack of awareness amongst the nurses interviewed about the importance of good communication with patients. This was coupled with an absence of organisational systems to develop information pathways and limited understanding of relevant tests by staff. Some patients adopted the role of passive patient and trusted staff to make decisions for them; however, passivity was exacerbated by deficient dissemination of information by nurses. Such deficiencies both detract from the individual's ability to be a partner in care and also emphasise a culture that does not appear to be serious about partnership with patients.

The study highlights that information giving to in-patients undergoing diagnostic investigations has been neglected. Analysis of the data supports the need and wishes of patients to receive information. The respondents in the study all recognised that there was a gap in providing specific and timely information.

Nurses spend a considerable proportion of their time in direct patient contact and the giving of information is an integral component in nursing care.

This study has challenged an aspect of information giving in a ward environment in order to deliver quality care. All nurses ended the interview by stating that they would change their practice to ensure that they gave information about investigations promptly to patients. The interviews encouraged the respondents to think about their current practice and how they could implement change.

Part 2
Relatives' and carers' experience of accessing information about their family member, compared with the perception of nurses regarding their practice of information giving
Debbie Reynolds

Intention

This chapter examines:

- How nurses ascertain the information needs of the carer
- Who the carer approaches for information and how useful they found the information
- Nurses' perceptions of information giving to carers
- Factors that hinder communication between nurse and carer

The term 'carer' is used throughout for brevity. This collective term should be considered as including all persons on whom the patient may be dependent after discharge.

Introduction

The interaction of staff with carers is often significant in facilitating the patient's journey. Such communication has been reported in the literature as lacking; and sharing of information between nurses and carers is too frequently ineffective. This study explores the experience of carers when seeking information, and compares their experiences with the perception of nursing staff regarding their practice of sharing information with carers.

Background

The researcher is a Patient Care Coordinator working within elderly medicine at a district general hospital. This role is concerned with improving the patients' journey by ensuring there are no delays in treatment and diagnosis. An important aspect of the role is ensuring that the patient and carer are aware of the plan of treatment and likely length of stay.

The researcher had noted deficits in communication between staff and carers in the clinical areas for which she was responsible. Reflection on this personal experience led to the development of a study to explore a problem that occurred regularly and had potentially serious consequences.

Key literature review

Literature reviewed prior to commencing the study highlighted that carers' perception of their role in relation to the patient was not understood; and understanding this role was crucial to determining their information (Aranda and Peerson, 2001; Cawthra, 1999).

Nurses do not always acknowledge the contribution that carers can make to the patient journey. It is reported that, depending on how carers are perceived by professionals, the information they receive will be affected (Morris and Thomas 2002; Allen, 2000; Dewar *et al.*, 2003). These findings suggest that, in order for nurses to improve communication with carers, they need to acquire a deeper understanding of the role of the carer, and the impact that receiving information will have on the dynamics of the relationship between nurse/carer/patient.

Studies have demonstrated that carers have particular information needs. These include receiving accurate, specific information about diagnosis, prognosis and treatment (Ahrens, 2003; Van der Smagt-Duijnstee *et al.*, 2001; Morris and Thomas, 2002) and information that was truthful (Norton *et al.*, 2003; Van der Smagt-Duijnstee *et al.*, 2001). Contemporary government directives also acknowledge the contribution of carers to the NHS (Health and Social Care Act, 2001; Department of Health, 2001a; Kennedy, 2001).

The literature acknowledges that lack of information is a cause of stress and anxiety to carers (Morris and Thomas, 2002; Bailey and Mion, 1997). Barriers to communication that exacerbate dissatisfaction for carers include inadequate time, lack of understanding of the carer's needs, and an inconsistent team approach (Ahrens, 2003; Mi-kuen *et al.*, 1999). The approach, attitudes and knowledge of the staff were also factors that affected communication (De Lucio *et al.*, 2000; Stedt-Kurki *et al.*, 2001).

Insufficient research exists to provide solutions in bridging the gap between the carers' expectations of receiving information and the current practice of nurses. The studies reviewed have predominantly been undertaken in specialist areas, which suggests that research within general acute areas is indicated.

The study

The study sought to explore, from the perspective of the carer, the experience of obtaining information about a patient for whom they were caring. This data was compared to nurses' perception of communicating with carers. The aim of the study was, therefore, to identify whether a gap existed between the carers' experience and the nurses' perception.

A retrospective qualitative design was selected, which enabled the researcher to gain insight into the lived experiences of the respondents (Polit and Hungler, 1997; Parahoo, 1997). By exploring the experience of carers and nurses, the researcher gained a deep understanding of the process of information exchange. This understanding ensured that the recommendations were firmly grounded within the experiences of nurses and carers.

The research was carried out on a medical ward for older people in a district general hospital. The data collection was carried out using a two-stage approach. Interviews were selected as the primary data collection tool. The interview, enabled a deeper level of data to be generated and, permitted the researcher to explore specific issues raised by respondents. The telephone interview was selected, in preference to face-to-face interviews, as the most suitable method for data collection from carers. The researcher undertook all interviews.

The sample comprised:

- Five carers of patients who had been cared for on a medical ward for older people
- Five qualified nurses working on the same ward as where carers had been recruited

Stage I

The first stage consisted of semi-structured telephone interviews with carers regarding the experience of obtaining information. The telephone interview limits the inconvenience to respondents and was more manageable within the logistics of the study.

The five interviews carried out with carers generated a rich data set. The interview asked the respondents a range of questions focusing on the sort of information they had wanted when the person for whom they were caring was in hospital. The semi-structured approach to the interview allowed respondents to raise many associated issues and concerns that might not have emerged through, for example, a questionnaire (Bryman, 2001; Parahoo, 1997).

Carers were interviewed retrospectively, after the discharge of the patient from hospital. Retrospective studies are criticised for being subjective, as the respondent is relying on memory of the events and may be selective in viewing the past (Parahoo, 1997). The researcher felt that interviewing carers whilst the patient was still hospitalised might have caused unnecessary stress and generated biased responses. Carers might have felt inhibited about being critical out of concern for retribution by the care team. They might have either declined the invitation to participate or not given honest accounts of their experiences. The researcher considered that, even though the participants might have forgotten the details of certain events or be selective in their accounts, they would still have an overall impression of the experience and any important events would still be significant.

Stage 2

The second stage involved five face-to-face semi-structured interviews with nurses, using open-ended questions, to explore their perceptions regarding their practice of giving information to carers. Through the interviews nurses explored their experience of giving information to carers. The interview was an opportunity to reflect and consider ways of improving their practice and enhancing nursing care based on previous experiences. As for the carers, the retrospective interview was considered an appropriate method for this study.

Findings

The common themes that emerged were that the quality of information was important, and that carers and nurses need to have access to each other in order for effective communication to happen. Carers demonstrated that they had a legitimate role and considered themselves to be 'experts' about the person for whom they were caring. The need for staff to be truthful was also highlighted.

Quality of information

Carers expected information to be timely, consistent, free from jargon and sufficient for them to understand the medical plan, diagnosis and prognosis; this is supported by the literature (Ahrens, 2003; Van der Smagt-Duijnstee, 2001; Morris and Thomas, 2002). The need for information was greatest on admission and in the days that followed. Jamerson *et al.* (1996) describe this experience as 'hovering', an initial sense of confusion, stress and uncertainty. Information seeking is a tactic to move beyond the 'hovering state' and to identify the patient's progress (Jamerson *et al.*, 1996).

Many carers felt that they did not receive adequate information and this resulted in the development of a poor nurse–carer relationship and dissatisfaction with the quality of care. Andershed and Ternestedt (1998) described carer involvement as either 'being in the light' or 'being in the dark'. 'Being in the light' described a trusting relationship based on mutual benefit between carer and staff. 'Being in the dark' was where insufficient interplay and collaboration existed and carers were not seen as important or acknowledged by the staff. Similar studies also considered negative and positive experiences from the perspective of carers (Main, 2002; Attree, 2001; Lloyd, 2000).

Nurses acknowledged that communication with carers was pivotal to their role, a view supported by Miller *et al.* (2001). However, as in De Lucio *et al.*'s (2000) study, some nurses found exchanging information to be stressful and anxiety-provoking. Carers experienced difficulties when nurses disclosed bad news, used complex language and did not recognise non-verbal cues, which is comparable with the findings of Chauhan and Long (2000). Although McCulloch (2004) found that patients were satisfied with the language used, she also identified a deficit in recognising the non-verbal aspects of communication.

Staff were comfortable with disclosure and discussion about resuscitation. This response is in contrast with studies undertaken with general nurses, which have often reported that this area of communication is difficult (Main, 2002). Positive responses could be related to clear guidelines and policies, and training at the NHS Trust. All the nurses interviewed worked with older people, and, consequently, the sample may have been skewed in favour of those nurses who had greater opportunity to have such discussions

However, nurses expressed difficulty with discussing a diagnosis without additional information to guide them. This may indicate that the nurses in the study practiced within a medical model and believed that such disclosure remains the responsibility of medical doctors. These findings were similar to those identified by Martin (1998), who found that ritual action appeared to underpin nurse responses regarding the power of medical doctors, information giving and disclosure.

Conversely, the study demonstrated that carers considered information from the medical doctors to be more credible than from nurses. The information that carers received from medical doctors was judged to be of greater value, even if the nurses had already offered the same information. Nurses were able to give accurate information with the same level of detail as medical staff, but carers were reassured by the ritualistic practice of receiving information from medical doctors; this is comparable to Biley and Wright's (1997) findings. It is acknowledged within the literature that nurses taking over work previously done by medical doctors is increasing (Dowling *et al.*, 1995; Dowling *et al.*, 1996), and therefore blurring of the boundaries between medicine and nursing is likely to continue and lead to further difficulties with role responsibilities.

Accessibility

Accessing staff, identifying the relevant person, and the attitude of some nurses affected the way in which carers received information. This is supported by Main (2002), who argues that carers should receive consistent information from staff who are familiar to them, who are approachable and with whom they have a rapport.

Nurses and carers both cited time constraints as reasons for inadequate communication. Although nurses saw communication as pivotal to their role, they seldom allowed it to take priority within their working day. As the pace of health care has changed it seems that the way a shift is organised has not. Nurses need to think smarter and work differently (Huber, 2000; Girvin, 1998). The studies undertaken by Medland (1998) and Bailey and Mion (1997) demonstrate that by rearranging the way nurses communicate with carers and by acting in a more proactive way, satisfaction levels can be increased for nurses, carers and patients.

Nurses had differing opinions on the type of information they were happy to discuss. Respondents frequently mentioned the dilemma of disclosure of information, particularly by telephone, and their duty of care towards the patient regarding disclosure. The lack of clarity regarding telephone disclosure highlights a lack of awareness of local policies and procedures, which could reflect leadership or accountability issues. Therefore nurses not only have a responsibility to gain the knowledge needed to practice, but also require good leadership to help to identify the gaps in knowledge (Huber, 2000).

Nurses reported difficulty dealing with conflict and managing 'difficult' carers. Massucci (2000) describes being a 'difficult relative' as an involuntary response to being helpless as a loved one suffers. Nurses need to gain a greater insight into the behaviour and lived experience of carers, as well as acquiring a better understanding of conflict management.

'Expert' carers

Responses from carers demonstrated that they had a positive contribution to make, had a role within the delivery of care, and that they also needed to be cared for (Greenwood, 1998; Lloyd, 2000; Allen, 2000). Nurses acknowledged the rights of the carers and some saw a connection to their importance and role. The findings suggest that greater emphasis needs to be placed on the valuable contribution that carers can make and the need for nurses to establish a rapport with carers; a view supported by Bailey and Mion (1997) and Allen (2000).

Lundh (2001) highlights the need for professionals to put to one side their existing preconceptions and to be more open to what carers are saying. Patients need holistic care, and that has to include all those involved in caring for them. The Human Rights Act (1998), article 8, states that everyone has a right to respect for his private and family life; this must extend to when a patient is admitted to hospital. Patients are part of a family and social network that does not disappear when admitted to hospital (Binnie and Titchen, 1999).

Cawood (2001) found that 100% of carers thought they were entitled to know 'most' or 'all' of the information regarding the person for whom they were caring, and 75% thought they were still entitled to this even if the patient was opposed to any member of the family being informed. Adopting the right level of disclosure was a concern for many nurses. The Code of Professional Conduct (Nursing and Midwifery Council, 2002a) states that confidentiality must be protected. If the patient is unable to consent then a decision to disclose must be made on the basis of what is considered to be in the patient's best interests. Although the guidance for staff is clear, in practice it is not so easy for staff to address, and a consistent approach may not be adopted.

Truth

There was a good level of consistency between carers, nurses and literature in relation to truthfulness. Carers highlighted the need to build up a rapport with staff and the need for truthful and honest communication, even if the news was not good. Norton *et al.* (2003) and Van der Smagt-Duijnstee *et al.* (2001) identified similar findings. Nurses agreed that truth and trust were essential to the relationship between staff and carers, a view supported by Day and Stannard (1999).

Recommendations

Ward managers need to identify knowledge gaps regarding effective communication and identify individual learning needs as part of personal development plans. A competency-based educational programme needs to be established which incorporates communication skills (with an emphasis on breaking bad news), management of conflict, disclosure of information and confidentiality. Wards need to adopt a unified approach to telephone disclosure to ensure that nurses fulfil their responsibilities regarding the code of professional conduct.

To improve the exchange of information and involvement of carers at an early stage in the patient's journey, the ward manager needs to establish a proactive approach to time management. This could be achieved by introducing a programme of contacting carers at an agreed time on a regular basis to update them on the patient's progress and discuss the care planned. Such an approach would ensure that nurses involve carers at an early stage and allows carers to establish rapport with a named individual. A robust system needs to be established which will identify a named person for carers to contact. In conjunction with this, a review of the effectiveness of the named nurse system needs to be undertaken.

An assessment of carers' needs must be included as part of the patient assessment and the carers' preferred involvement in the delivery of care must be included in the care plan. Nurses need to be encouraged to consider the 'role' that carers have during a hospital admission and acknowledge the positive contribution that they can make.

Implications

Failure to implement the recommendations will lead to continued frustration on the part of carers and nurses. Lack of consistent, honest, timely information will continue to result in misunderstanding and breakdown in the nurse–carer relationship and will perpetuate negative outcomes. Implementing the recommendations of this study will address the gap between the carer's expectations and current practice. This will result in improved patient care, effective communication, greater job satisfaction and positive relationships with patients and their carers.

Conclusion

The study demonstrated that carers have a very definite view about their right to receive information. Although it was encouraging that some carers were very satisfied with the information they received, were included in discussions and were very satisfied with the relationship they had with the ward staff, it was disappointing that other carers had very unsatisfactory experiences.

Nurses acknowledged the importance of effective communication and the need for it to be pivotal to their role, and areas of good practice were identified. However, working with carers was not recognised as an integral role of the nurse and built into workload models. This was exacerbated by a lack of consistent argument concerning the degree to which the carer should be seen as a holistic part of the caring process; either having valuable contributions to make, or legitimately needing to be 'cared for' themselves.

The study demonstrates that a gap between carers' expectations and the practice of exchanging information exists and has a detrimental effect on the relationship between carer and nurse. The study has given nurses the opportunity to reflect on their practice and to consider how they could implement change for the benefit of patients, carers and themselves.

Part 3
Common partnership themes
Peter J. Martin

Introduction

Eastbrook and Reynolds have presented two papers that explore different perspectives of information giving. Eastbrook's work focuses on information giving between patients and nurses; and Reynolds focuses on information giving between carers and nurses. The studies are comparable in the approach taken to the subject. Despite coming from different perspectives, both papers offer remarkably similar insights into this important aspect of nursing care. The findings indicate that nursing staff poorly managed information giving in relation to patients and carers.

Research design

The aim of Eastbrook's and Reynolds' studies was to explore how nurses and patients/carers perceived current practice in information giving and receiving. The studies both adopt a primarily qualitative design, which is congruent with the intention to explore 'information giving'. By engaging both nurses and patients/carers, Eastbrook's and Reynolds' research is at the partnership interface. The studies permit differences to be established in what nurses think they are doing and how the actions of nurses are perceived by patients/carers.

The research method used is similar, with both researchers using semi-structured interviews to collect data from patients or carers and qualified nursing staff. Eastbrook undertakes her interviews face-to-face and Reynolds uses a combination of face-to-face and telephone interviews. The studies are both small-scale and exploratory in nature. Eastbrook interviewed eight patients and seven staff and Reynolds interviewed five carers and five staff. The sequential nature of data collection allowed the researchers to examine 'real world' problems of partnership that had arisen for patients/carers with the nurses who were interviewed.

Findings

Eastbrook's and Reynolds' papers examine the nature of partnership though the exchange of information within a health care setting. The key assumption underpinning the papers is that the health care professional and the patient/carer should share information in an unhindered manner. Partnership is, therefore, enhanced through striving to improve the flow of information between parties in the health care system. This assumption is untested within the current studies; however, both papers cite literature in support or literature demonstrating the consequence of poor information exchange. Furthermore, improving the quality and quantity of information available to patients and carers is the focus or underpinning message of many recent NHS documents (Department of Health, 2000, 2001b).

An analysis of the papers by Eastbrook and Reynolds identifies the recurring themes of communication, confidence and culture. These themes are interrelated; the culture of the environment impacts upon the confidence of the nurse, which inhibits or enhances his or her ability to communicate with patients or carers. In each of these areas the flow of information can be impeded or enhanced.

Communication

Eastbrook and Reynolds do not, within the scope of the papers, differentiate between 'communication' and 'information giving'. The studies focus on verbal, rather than written, information, and nurses engage in verbal communication in order to relay specific information to patients and carers. Thus, whilst the authors use the terms interchangeably, information giving is apparently embedded within communication. Neither paper adopts a position as to whether 'information giving' should be considered a nurse's role. Eastbrook does, however, note that nurses were reported as not taking ownership of information giving by any of her informants.

At a theoretical level communication is a fundamental medium by which nursing care is delivered (see Peplau, 1988; Orem, 1991; Watson, 1988 and others). The competence of the nurse to practically engage in effective communication is also a requirement of the Nursing and Midwifery Council for entry onto the register. Under the heading of care delivery, the nurse must demonstrate that he or she can effectively interact with a degree of fluency and spontaneity that makes information sharing with patients/clients and their relatives and colleagues possible (Nursing and Midwifery Council, 2002b). The nurses in Eastbrook and Reynolds should, therefore, be able to demonstrate both competence in communicating and a cognitive awareness of the importance of communicating.

The exchange of information is accomplished within a 'process of communicating' or as a 'product of communicating'. The nurses in the study engaged in both 'communicating' and 'passing information', which may be regarded as two different pursuits. Information was exchanged primarily as a task, but this may be a weakness within the design. Nurses may not have expounded upon the complex interpersonal skills in which they engaged, because the researchers were interested in information giving. Similarly, in the studies the focus of the information giving related primarily to medical intervention of some form rather than discussion of nursing interventions. However, nurses, as part of the multi-disciplinary team, should be able to relay accurate information as required or make suitable referral to someone more able.

The nurses in Eastbrook's and Reynolds' studies appeared to regard information giving primarily as a product for which time must be allocated within the work schedule. Both Eastbrook's and Reynolds' samples refer to information giving being hampered by time constraints and staffing levels. This suggests that either there was a poor level of general communication taking place in the clinical environments or that 'information giving' was perceived as a discrete function separate from nurse–patient or nurse–carer interactions. Information giving as a task discrete from general communication can be a duty to be achieved in terms of quantity rather than quality. The nurse may give the required quantity of information without achieving quality. For example 'nil by mouth' is a specific and clear instruction. However, the patient may be left confused and anxious about the implications of such an instruction and fall prey to the fantasies and anxieties described by Wilson-Barnett (1990). It must be assumed that there were many examples of good communication between nurses, patients and carers. However, Eastbrook's and Reynolds' work emphasises areas of ineffective communication reported by carers and patients.

The two studies suggest that communication in the direction of patient to nurse and carer to nurse was also reported as problematic. Eastbrook's study indicated that some patients were passive in relation to seeking information; and Reynolds' carers did not trust the information given to them by nurses and placed nurses in an uncomfortable position with regard to disclosure. These problems appear to stem from the consequences of the problems nurses were reporting. In each case the problem was within the communication process rather than with the carer or patient. For example, carers may have more confidence in information received from a 'confident' medical doctor than a nurse who demonstrably lacks confidence in the information he or she is providing.

The patient and carer, as the recipient of care and information, were critical of the nurse's ability and timeliness in communicating information. However, the patients in these studies were receiving information about tests and carers about prognosis. In some instances nurses might offer information at a time when patients or carers were unable to process the information through anxiety, pain or information overload. Nurses might have felt that information had been given, but have failed to ensure that it had been received.

The nurses in Eastbrook's and Reynolds' papers asserted that communicating with patients and carers was important, but this did not appear to be demonstrated in practice. Providing patients and carers with information was not placed within a framework of more general communication with patients and carers. The nurses in the study presented Eastbrook and Reynolds with many practical reasons why they did not share information, which may suggest that the nurses considered it less important than other tasks. The nurses in Reynolds' study described anxiety associated with communicating to carers that may also lead to avoidance of communicating. The two behaviours reported in these studies may be related: a link between task-oriented behaviour and avoiding patient contact has been reported elsewhere (Menzies Lyth, 1959).

The nurses in the study did not appear to recognise the significance of communication with patients/carers as an aspect of nursing care or as a specific function in the delivery of good nursing care. The findings of these papers indicate that poor communication weakened any sense of partnership between nurses and patients/carers.

Confidence

In order for nurses to communicate information to patients and carers in an effective manner they must feel confident in their ability to do so. Eastbrook's and Reynolds' papers suggest that nurses may be reluctant to communicate information effectively to patients and carers through lack of confidence.

Confidence may stem from the nurse's lack of knowledge about a particular medical test or procedure. Where a patient or carer seeks information about an unusual procedure, the nurse's reticence may be understandable. Reluctance to discuss a procedure that the nurse is unfamiliar with is commendable and proper. However, where the information requested relates to a procedure undertaken regularly within the clinical environment the nurse's knowledge is deficient. The Nursing and Midwifery Council Code of Conduct, to which nurses adhere, obliges the nurse to maintain the currency of his or her knowledge and skills (Nursing and Midwifery Council, 2004, paragraph 6). The nurse may be reported to the Nursing and Midwifery Council for disciplinary action if his or her behaviour falls outside of that which is acceptable under this Code of Conduct. Similarly, the competencies for registration require that the nurse demonstrate commitment to continuing professional development and personal supervision activities (Nursing and Midwifery Council, 2002a). If nurses are to provide patients/carers with timely and accurate information they must first furnish themselves with appropriate knowledge and understanding in order to discharge this responsibility. However, nurses in the studies indicated that the practical problems to do with workload and time often got in the way of giving information to patients and carers.

Confidence may also relate to the environment in which the nurse works. Study participants indicated that they did not have a sense of ownership of information giving and were not motivated to locate information. This did not suggest a team approach to facilitating the patient journey. Much health care is delivered through the multi-professional team, with all members of the team working in a collegiate manner to the benefit of the patient. However, in some areas, teams are not fully developed and patients receive the attentions of the individual professionals concurrently, but not collectively. This compartmentalised activity compromises communication between all members of the health care team, and consequently impacts upon the flow of information to patients and carers.

Eastbrook's nurse participants reported that they thought patients and carers would derive information about complex clinical procedures through the media. The range of good quality information available to patients through the media and Internet is an important and significant development in the last decade. It has resulted in a generally better informed and discerning consumer of health care. However, this finding seems to indicate a perceived lowering of professional status amongst nurses in the sample. Participants seemed to imply that information giving by nurses was redundant because patients accessed information from alternative sources. This may explain the lowly perception of the importance of information giving expressed by the nurse participants.

Confidence in information giving, amongst Eastbrook's and Reynolds' participants, appeared to relate to where nurses did not understand the information, did not have access to all the information or did not consider that it was their job to relay the information. Eastbrook's and Reynolds' work suggests that partnership increases with the confidence of those involved within the partnership. Increasing confidence leads to clearer, more complete and more assertive communication.

Culture

The culture of the environment will impact upon the quality of the communication. Eastbrook's and Reynolds' work suggests a number of areas where culture has impacted upon practice. Eastbrook cites Redwood's reference to the passive patient as the ideal patient, an expression of a culture that may persist within the environments from which Eastbrook and Reynolds drew their samples. Maintaining patients in a passive state may manifest itself as a desire not to 'frighten' or 'confound' patients with too much detail. Hence nurses will give minimum information and reassurances that the patient/carer should not worry. Such reassurances were recognised by nurses as being detrimental as early as Nightingale (1992, p. 58):

> They [patients] don't want you [nurses] to be lachrymose and whining with them, they like you to be fresh and active and interested, but they cannot bear absence of mind, and they are so tired of the advise and preaching they receive from every body, no matter whom it is, they see.

The nurse may also be over-familiar with the structure and processes within the clinical environment and forget to tell patients what they need to know, assuming it is already known. Such careless omission of detail is a manifestation of poor communication, but is also influenced by an environment where communication is focused on inter-professionalism at the expense of effective communication to patients and carers. Communication is hierarchical with the patient/carer being the least significant component of the communication chain.

Establishing and maintaining patients in a passive position in the health care system is a demonstration of the exercise of power. Nurses reportedly chose not to give all the information to patients because, as a consequence, they may be asked questions which they could not answer. The nurses in the samples appeared to find difficulty in defining the limits of their knowledge to patients. This may be a response to ongoing stress without adequate support and consequent 'burnout'; it may also be a protection of professional status within a culture where status is seen as valued (Benner and Wrubel, 1989, p. 385):

> The hallmark of the expert nurse is the recognition of her or his strengths and weaknesses and the ability to shape her or his practice towards strengths.

An alternative interpretation may be that, in seeking further information to address patient questions, work is generated for a stretched nursing team. Whichever interpretation is accepted the consequence is the reduced likelihood of being able to establish mutually beneficial partnerships with patients or carers. This may be evidenced by the mistrust shown by Reynolds' carers to the information given to them by nurses.

Power relations underpin health care systems and the environments from which Eastbrook and Reynolds samples were drawn appear to be no different. A culture based on collaborative working provides a good context for partnerships; this was not evidenced in the two papers. The culture appeared to emphasise hierarchy and status, with patients and carers being given information in an apathetic, reluctant manner.

Conclusion

From Eastbrook's and Reynolds' papers three important facets of partnership have been highlighted. The ongoing use of effective communication between nurses and patients/carers provided a context for transmitting essential information. Without this context, information giving becomes a task to be achieved that may be forgotten, poorly delivered or actively avoided. In order to communicate effectively, nurses needed to feel confident in their knowledge base and in their ability to communicate the information. Finally, both confidence and communication were influenced by the culture in which the nurse worked. Where the culture was hierarchical nurses appeared less confident or able to deliver necessary information to patients and carers.

If mutually beneficial partnerships are to flourish, Eastbrook's and Reynolds' studies suggest that the culture should be one of equality where nurses, patients and carers work together to the benefit of the patient. Such a culture requires nurses to engage with patients and carers in an honest and open manner without recourse to professional status. It also requires nurses to consider how communication underpins the delivery of nursing care and be more conscious and aware of its use in everyday practice.

References

Ahrens, T. (2003) Improving communications at the end of life: implications for length of stay in an Intensive Care Unit and resource use. *American Journal of Critical Care*, **2**(4), 317–28.

Allen, D. (2000) Negotiating the role of expert carers on an adult hospital ward. *Sociology of Health and Illness*, **22**(2), 149–71.

American Academy of Orthopaedic Surgeons (1996) Patients need more information. *Bulletin*, **44**(1) (http://www2.aaos.org/aaos/archives/bulletin/jan96/info.htm).

Andershed, B. and Ternestedt, B. (1998) Involvement of carers in the care of the dying in different care cultures: Involvement in the Dark or in the Light? *Cancer Nursing*, **21**(2), 106–111.

Aranda, S. and Peerson, A. (2001) Caregiving in advanced cancer: lay decision making. *Journal of Palliative Care*, **17**(4), 270–7.

Arthur, V. (1995) Written patient information: a review of the literature. *Journal of Advanced Nursing*, **21**(6), 1081–6.

Attree, M. (2001) Patients' and carers' experiences and perspectives of good and not so good quality care. *Journal of Advanced Nursing*, **33**(4), 456–66.

Audit Commission (1993) *What Seems to Be the Matter: Communication Between Hospitals and Patients*. Audit Commission, London

Bailey, D. and Mion, L. (1997) Improving care giver's satisfaction with information received during hospitalisation. *Journal of Nursing Administration*, **27**(1), 21–7.

Benner, P. and Wrubel, J. (1989) *The Primacy of Caring*. Addison-Wesley, Menlo Park, CA.

Biley, F. and Wright, S. (1997) Towards a defence of nursing routine and ritual. *Journal of Clinical Nursing*, **6**(2), 115–19.

Binnie, A. and Titchen, A. (1999) *Freedom to Practice: the Development of Patient-centred Nursing*. Butterworth-Heinemann, Oxford.

Breisch, L. (1999) Motivate! *Nursing Management Chicago*, **30**(3), 27–9.

Bryman, A. (2001) *Social Research Methods*. Oxford University Press, New York.

Cable, S., Lumsdaine, J. and Semple, M. (2003) Informed consent. *Nursing Standard*, **18**(12), 47–58.

Caress, A. (2003) Giving information to patients. *Nursing Standard*, **17**(43), 47–54.

Cawood, T. (2001) Great expectations: a carer dilemma. *British Medical Journal*, **323**(7325), 1375.

Cawthra, L. (1999) Older people's health information needs. *Health Libraries Review*, **16**, 97–105.

Chauhan, G. and Long, A. (2000) Communication is the essence of nursing: ethical foundations. *British Journal of Nursing*, **9**(15), 979–85.

Clements, H. and Melby, V. (1998) An investigation into the information obtained by patients undergoing gastroscopy investigations. *Journal of Clinical Nursing*, **7**(4), 333–42.

Cormack, D. (1996) *The Research Process in Nursing*. Blackwell Science, London.

Cortis, J. and Lacey, A. (1995) Measuring the quality and quantity of information-giving to in-patients. *Journal of Advanced Nursing*, **24**, 674–81.

Coulter, A., Entwistle, V. and Gilbert, D. (1999) Sharing decisions with patients: is the information good enough? *British Medical Journal*, **318**, 318–22.

Day, L. and Stannard, D. (1999) Developing trust and connection with patients and their families. *Critical Care Nurse*, **19**(3), 66–71.

De Lucio, L., Lopez, F., Lopez, M., Hesse, B. and Vaz, M. (2000) Training programme in techniques of self-control and communication skills to improve nurses' relationships with carers of seriously ill patients: a randomised controlled study. *Journal of Advanced Nursing*, **32**(2), 425–31.

Dewar, B., Tocher, R. and Watson, W. (2003) Enhancing partnerships with carers in care settings. *Nursing Standard*, **17**(40), 33.

Department of Health (2000) *The NHS Plan: a Plan for Investment, a Plan for Reform*. Department of Health, London.

Department of Health (2001a) *National Service Framework for Older People*. Department of Health, London.

Department of Health (2001b) *The Expert Patient: a New Approach to Chronic Disease Management for the 21st Century*. Department of Health, London.

Dowling, S., Barrett, S. and West, R. (1995) With nurse practitioners, who needs house officers? *British Medical Journal*, **311**(7000), 309–13.

Dowling, S., Martin, R., Skidmore, P., Doyal, l., Cameron, A. and Lloyd, S. (1996) Nurses taking on junior doctors' work: a confusion of accountability. *British Medical Journal*, **312**(7040), 1211–14.

Duxbury, J. (2000) *Difficult Patients*. Butterworth-Heinemann, Oxford.

Gert, H. (2002) Avoiding surprises: a model for informing patients. *Hastings Centre Report*, **32**(5), 23–32.

Girvin, J. (1998) *Leadership and Nursing*. Macmillan, Basingstoke.

Greenwood, J. (1998) Meeting the needs of patients' carers. *Professional Nurse*, **14**(3), 156–7.

Greenwood, J. (2002) Employing a range of methods to meet patient information needs. *Professional Nurse*, **18**(4), 233–6.

Health and Social Care Act (2001) http://www.hmso.gov.uk/acts/acts2001.

House, A. and Stark, D. (2002) Anxiety in medical patients. *British Medical Journal*, **325**(7357), 207–9.

Huber, D. (2000) *Leadership and Nursing Care Management*, 2nd edn. W. B. Saunders, Pennsylvania.

Hughes, S. (2002) The effects of giving patients pre-operative information. *Nursing Standard*, **16**(28), 33–7.

Human Rights Act (1998) `http://www.opsi.gov.uk/acts/acts1998/80042-d.htm#sch1`.

Jamerson, P., Scheibmeir, M., Bott, M., Crighton, F., Hinton, R. and Cobb, A. (1996) The experiences of families with a carer in the intensive care unit. *Heart and Lung*, **25**(6), 467–74.

Jensen, J. (1987) Most physicians believe patients obtain healthcare information from mass media. *Modern Healthcare Chicago*, **17**(19), 110–11.

Kessels, R. (2003) Patient's memory for medical information. *Journal of the Royal Society of Medicine*, **96**(5), 219.

Kennedy, I. (2001) *Learning from Bristol – the Report of the Public Enquiry into Children's Heart Surgery at the Bristol Royal Infirmary 1984–1995*. Department of Health, London.

Kinrade, S. (2002) Communication breakdown. *Nursing Times*, **98**(3), 40–1.

Le Tourneau, B. (2004) Physicians and nurses: friends or foes. *Journal of Healthcare Management*, **49**(1), 12–15.

Lloyd, L. (2000) Caring about the carers: only half the picture? *Critical Social Policy*, **20**(1), 136–50.

Lundh, U. (2001) Impact of professional carers of structured interviews with families. *British Journal of Nursing*, **10**(10), 677–82.

Main, J. (2002) Management of carers of patients who are dying. *Journal of Clinical Nursing*, **11**(6), 794–801.

Martin, G. (1998) Ritual action and its effect on the role of the nurse as advocate. *Journal of Advanced Nursing*, **27**(1), 189–94.

Massucci, L. (2000) Lessons from the other side. *Nursing*, **30**(5), 9.

Mayberry, M. and Mayberry, J. (2001) Towards better informed consent in endoscopy: a study of information and consent processes in gastroscopy and flexible sigmoidoscopy. *European Journal of Gastroenterology and Hepatology*, **13**(12), 1467–76.

McColl, E., Thomas, L. and Bond, S. (1996) A study to determine patient satisfaction with nursing care. *Nursing Standard*, **10**(52), 34–8.

McIntosh, A. and Shaw, C. (2002) Barriers to patient information provision in primary care: patients' and general practitioners' experiences and expectations of information for low back pain. *Health Expectations*, **6**, 19–29.

McCulloch, P. (2004) The patient experience of receiving bad news from health professionals. *Professional Nurse*, **19**(5), 1–5.

Medland, J. (1998) Effectiveness of a structured communication program for family members of patients in an ICU. *American Journal of Critical Care*, **7**(1), 24–36.

Menzies Lyth, I. (1959) The functioning of social systems as a defence against anxiety. In: *Containing Anxiety in Institutions: Selected Essays* (ed. I. Menzies Lyth (1988)). Free Association Books, London.

Mi-kuen, T., French, P. and Kai-kwong, L. (1999) The needs of the family of critically ill neurosurgical patients: a comparison of nurses' and family members' perceptions. *Journal of Neuroscience Nursing*, **31**(6), 348–56.

Miller, E., Deets, C. and Miller, R. (2001) Nurse call and the work environment: lessons learned. *Journal of Nursing Care Quality*, **15**(3), 7–16.

Mills, M. and Sullivan, K. (1999) The importance of information giving for patients newly diagnosed with cancer: a review of the literature. *Journal of Clinical Nursing*, **8**, 631–42.

Mordiffi, S., Tan, S. and Wong, M. (2003) Information provided to surgical patients versus information needed. *AORN Journal*, **77**(3), 546–62.

Morris, S. and Thomas, C. (2002) The need to know: informal carers and information. *European Journal of Cancer Care*, **11**, 183–7.

Neuberger, J. and Tallis, R. (1999) Education and debate: do we need a new word for patients? *British Medical Journal*, **318**(7200), 1756–8.

Nicklin, J. (2002) Improving the quality of written information for patients. *Nursing Standard*, **16**(49), 39–44.

Nightingale, F. (1992) *Notes on Nursing*. Lippincott, Philadelphia.

NHS Executive (1999) *Clinical Governance: Quality in the NHS*. Department of Health, London.

Norton, S., Tilden, V., Tolle, V., Nelson, C. and Talamantes Eggman, S. (2003) Life support withdrawal: communication and conflict. *Journal of Critical Care*, **12**(6), 548–56.

Nursing and Midwifery Council (2002a) *Code of Professional Conduct*. Nursing and Midwifery Council, London.

Nursing and Midwifery Council (2002b) *Requirements for Pre-Registration Nursing Programmes Section 3 Nursing Competencies*. Nursing and Midwifery Council, London.

Nursing and Midwifery Council (2004) *The Nursing and Midwifery Council Code of Professional Conduct: Standards for Conduct, Performance and Ethics*. Nursing and Midwifery Council, London.

Orem, D. (1991) *Nursing: Concepts of Practice*. Mosby, St Louis.

Parahoo, K. (1997) *Nursing Research. Principles, Process and Issues*. Macmillan, Basingstoke.

Pediani, R. and Walsh, M. (1999) Changing practice: are memos the answer? *Nursing Standard*, **14**(24), 36–40.

Peplau, H. (1988) *Interpersonal Relations in Nursing*. Macmillan, London.

Polit, D. and Hungler, B. (1997) *Essentials of Nursing Research: Methods, Appraisal and Utilisation*, 4th edn. Lippincott, New York.

Price, B. (2004) Conducting sensitive patient interviews. *Nursing Standard*, **18**(38), 45–52.

Redwood, H. (2002) *Patient Education: the End of One-way Traffic*. Health and Age (http://www.healthandage.com/).

Stedt-Kurki, O., Paavilainen, E., Tammentie, T. and Paunonen-Ilmonen, M. (2001) Interaction between adult patients' family members and nursing staff on a hospital ward. *Scandinavian Journal of Caring Sciences*, **15**(2), 142–50.

Stevens, A. and Dowd, S. (1999) Patient education in nuclear medicine technology practice. *Journal of Nuclear Medicine Technology*, **27**(1), 4–14.

Scott, P., Valimaki, M., Leino-Kilpi, H. and Dassen, T. (2003) Autonomy, privacy and informed consent 1: Concepts and definitions. *British Journal of Nursing*, **12**(1), 43–7.

Van der Smagt-Duijnstee, M., Hamers, J., Huda, H. and Zuidhof, A. (2001) Carers of hospitalised stroke patients: their needs for information, counselling and accessibility. *Journal of Advanced Nursing*, **33**(3), 307–15.

Wallace, L. (1985) Surgical patients' preference for pre-operative information. *Patient Education and Counselling*, **7**, 377–87.

Watson, J. (1988) *Nursing: Human Science and Human Care*. National League for Nursing Press, New York.

White, E. (2002) Is information always good for patients? *Nursing Times*, **98**(3).

Wilson-Barnet, J. (1990) Diagnostic procedures. In: *Stress and Medical Procedures* (eds. M. Johnston and L. Wallace) Oxford University Press, New York.

Woodward, N. and Wallston, B. (1987) Age and health-care beliefs: self-efficacy as a mediator of low desire for control. *Psychology and Aging*, **2**, 3–8.

CHAPTER 5

Service partnerships

Introduction

Kimmy Eldridge

This section comprises three research reports and a critical review that extracts common themes relating to partnership working from the preceding papers. The three small-scale research studies were completed as part of a master's degree at the University of Essex:

- A phenomenological study into the experiences of critical care nurses working as part of a critical care outreach team by Elizabeth Carpenter
- Community stroke services research: a needs-based assessment by Moira Keating
- Initial assessments in community specialist palliative care: an evaluation of nurses' perceptions and experiences by Rachel Wilson

Carpenter's and Wilson's studies investigated how nurses felt working outside a team context. Keating's study is based on a multi-agency, corporate, needs-based assessment, to establish the services and support available to people who have suffered a stroke. All three researchers are experienced practising nurses in the area of their investigation.

Carpenter's paper is based on original research within three district general hospitals in which eight critical care outreach nurses were interviewed. Critical care nurses usually work in a highly technical and controlled environment and are seen as a clinical competent and elite workforce. These eight nurses had chosen to work in wards where the resources (staff expertise and equipment) were inadequate to support critically ill patients, resulting in patients being transferred to an intensive care unit. Carpenter explores factors that promote and hinder the outreach staff's integration into the ward team.

Keating's research took place in a specific borough and was funded jointly by a district general hospital, local social services, local community voluntary services, the local Stroke Association and a local advocacy scheme. The project thus had multi-agency ownership. Keating compared the discrepancies between demand for services expressed as wishes and the supply of services, including alternative perspectives of key agencies. The study employed questionnaires to survey service providers and users; both groups were also invited to focus group discussions.

Wilson's research was undertaken in a hospice setting. As an employing organisation and a care provider, the hospice views interdisciplinary assessment as the ideal model of assessment. Yet the reality of practice and resource pressure means that nurses inevitably carry out the assessment alone. Wilson sought to establish how nurses feel about performing the first assessment on their own without other members of the primary care team.

Part 1
A phenomenological study into the experiences of critical care nurses working as part of a critical care outreach team
Elizabeth C. Carpenter

Intention

- To examine the role of the critical care nurse as a member of an outreach team
- To identify factors that influence outreach team functioning

Introduction

Critical care services face significant challenges over the next decade. Although all aspects of care are under pressure, particular emphasis has been placed on the care of the acutely ill patient in secondary care. Overall, numbers of hospital in-patient beds are being reduced, and yet expectations are higher. For example, the case mix within hospitals over the next 5–10 years is set to become more complex, patient age is increasing, and patients often have multiple health problems (Stenhouse, 2001; Coombs and Dillon, 2002).

A body of work over the last few years has supported the view that critically ill patients in general ward areas are poorly served by the current
system (Goldhill *et al.*, 1999; McQuillan *et al.*, 1998; Franklin and Mathew,
1994) Perceived deficits in the care of the critically ill outside of the intensive care setting have been attributed to several factors. A number of studies
have identified higher morbidity or mortality in patients reported to have
received suboptimal management during the period before admission to
intensive care. The main causes are organisation failure, lack of knowledge,
failure to appreciate clinical urgency, lack of supervision and failure to seek
advice. McQuillan *et al.* (1998), Franklin and Mathew (1994), Chellel *et al.*
(2002) and Ball (2002) also identified that lack of basic nursing observation, patient assessment, problems of skill mix and workloads of ward staff
are other factors which affect performance. In addition, legislation relating to junior doctors' hours (the European Working Time Directive) has
reduced the experience level of trainee doctors and therefore the continuity
of patient care (Department of Health, 1991; Joint Consultants' Committee,
2002–2003).

Successive reforms, service reconfigurations and more flexible working have resulted in substantial changes in health care policy. (Department
of Health, 2000a, 2001a; Coombs and Dillon, 2002). The concept of critical care outreach received its first national airing in *Critical to Success*
(Audit Commission, 1999). The following year *Review of Comprehensive
Adult Critical Care* (Department of Health, 2000a) focused on the needs of
patients with potential or actual need for critical care based on the severity
of the illness, not where it was delivered. This system of care delivery was
seen as a way of reducing patient risk, intensive care admissions and the
high costs associated with intensive care. Critical care outreach nurses work
within small teams, independently and interdependently across professional
and speciality boundaries. However, little is known about their experiences.
The aim of this study was to explore the transition process and needs of
nurses moving away from critical care areas to work within outreach teams
in ward areas.

Background

As a senior intensive care nurse working within an Acute Trust that did not
have a critical care outreach team I felt there was a need to examine the experiences of members of these new outreach teams in order to inform future
planning and implementation of the outreach service.

The study

The study used phenomenology as an inductive research method (Omery, 1983) to investigate and describe the transition process and needs of nurses moving away from critical care areas to work within outreach teams. The objectives were to:

- Explore why critical care nurses become outreach team members
- Examine the experience of transition to the team and working on general wards
- Identify factors that promote and improve the practice of team members
- Identify factors that hinder their practice
- Identify the level of support that these nurses receive

The study employed non-probability, purposive sampling of eight (F and G grade) nurses currently working within critical care outreach teams (excluding line managers) within three district general hospitals. The rationale for excluding line managers working within teams was that it might have skewed results. Purposive sampling was adopted as it can be used to study the lived experiences of a specific population and collect exploratory data from an unusual population. It is used for in-depth, information-rich studies, when the population is highly unique and the sample hand-picked (Polit and Hungler, 1997; Bernard, 2000).

Data were collected through semi-structured taped interviews using an interview schedule. This was considered the most appropriate way to probe and explore meanings and interpretations (Edwards and Talbot, 1997) and allow the opportunity to follow new leads and obtain additional information through observation. Ethical approval was obtained from local research ethical committees and trust research departments.

Limitations of the study

The study sample was small, limiting generalisability to the population of outreach nurses in the United Kingdom. Although all members of individual teams were approached, time constraints prevented all members to be included in the study. The researcher was also known to some of the participants, which may have skewed the results. Attempts were made to bracket any preconceptions by the researcher so that the participants' experiences could be seen as they were. Three transcripts were examined by a senior colleague experienced in research, but the results of the study might have been more robust if all eight transcripts had been validated by independent analysis or the findings returned for verification to the participants. The time limit was a factor and confidentiality could not have been assured if the results of the transcripts were returned by post. The study used participants from three outreach teams across two regional health authorities. Therefore this study may serve as a foundation for future larger studies investigating whether outreach and interdisciplinary practice improves outcome management.

Findings

Four elements emerged from the data:

- Expectations of the role
- Support within the role
- Relationships
- Knowledge and skills

Expectations of the role

This element has four constituents: job satisfaction; independence; perceptions vs. reality of the role; and self-expectation.

Job satisfaction

Although most participants expressed some dissatisfaction with their previous role, those who had spent more than 10 years in critical care experienced less job satisfaction:

> I can do ITU standing on my head. You almost plop your brain out in the locker before you go on duty. You don't have to think about it. It was no longer a challenge.... It was the opportunity to do something brand new in an area I was very comfortable and confident in. (*nurse 8*)

Job satisfaction relates to individual need and the extent to which the job fulfils those needs. The participants experienced the need to look for new challenges within a familiar area of work. Studies by Cavanagh (1992) and Cartledge

(2001) identify that with regard to job dissatisfaction, lack of professional development, progress or achievement are seen as the dominant motivators, whilst pay is seen as a lower order motivator. This was identified by one participant:

> ... it wasn't the money, definitely not. It was the opportunity to do something brand new in an area I was very comfortable with. (*nurse 8*)

Stressful critical events within the outreach role appeared to give the majority of participants a high degree of job satisfaction:

> It was designed for me.... The critical thing, whether it be sick patients, trauma or cardiac arrest. (*nurse 7*)

Lally and Pearce (1996) support these findings and Sawatzky (1996) questions whether critical care attracts individuals who, by their disposition, tend to be more challenged than threatened by stressful situations. Korbasa (1982) takes this further and suggests that people who possess the attributes of hardiness are more likely to perceive stressors as a challenge rather than a threat. The development of hardiness is influenced by age, experience and personality and is a significant predictor of burnout (Lally and Pearce, 1996).

One individual expressed feelings of stress and burnout because of the nature of outreach work, and lack of support and commitment to the team, whilst being within a system over which the participant felt they had little control:

> I enjoyed outreach so much.... I don't feel quite the same now because of the whole drudge of it all and the same problems. It grinds you down. It's trying to play the teams to get the best for the patient. Get the patient in the right place, not pretend you can. 'Critical Care without Walls' is a load of rubbish. It thinks it is the politics and the doctors that don't accept outreach, I suppose. (*nurse 6*)

These findings concur with the findings of Keane *et al.* (1985).

Independence

The majority of participants felt that the role related to increased freedom, autonomy and responsibility with the opportunity to be innovative and creative:

> This thing was going to be ours, we could create it... (*nurse 2*)

> ... not being chained to a bed space... there's greater freedom now. (*nurse 1*)

These findings are consistent with studies on job satisfaction (Loher *et al.*, 1985; Ross and Reskin, 1992; Collins *et al.*, 2000).

Perceptions

It was clear that experienced critical care nurses felt that outreach gave them the opportunity to work more autonomously in a new way, whilst allowing them to challenge their knowledge and skills and further their professional development. Their preconceptions of the role were mostly at variance with the realities of working independently in an unknown environment and raised feelings of vulnerability in the majority of the participants:

> ... the cavalry has come out and it was quite a glorified position... (*nurse 2*)

The initial experience of working autonomously within an unfamiliar environment was seen as isolating and stressful for most intensive care team members:

> ... scared out of my wits.... I didn't have that safety net... that was quite a shock. (*nurse 4*)

It appeared less stressful for participants who had recent ward experience:

> I see things differently. I felt that I know this place like the back of my hand. (*nurse 7*)

Self-expectation

In the early stages of the role, most participants imposed high demands on themselves by trying to achieve unrealistic goals:

> ... we expected that we know everything... (*nurse 7*)

This often led to feelings of frustration and stress, although it became apparent that it was unrealistic:

> We know now you don't have to know everything. That lightened things really... yeah that was a very good point to get to... (*nurse 8*)

Support in the role

Support was considered the major 'facilitator' of the role and there were mixed views on whether participants felt supported. The constituent clusters to emerge in this element were primarily: team leadership; support within the team; and medical commitment and support.

Team leadership

The participants experienced different types of team leadership, through their line management, either inside or outside of their teams. Different leadership styles greatly influenced participants' feelings of empowerment:

> ... the team has always been self winding. (*nurse 5*)

Those participants who felt empowered identified that their manager afforded them trust and respect, and gave them opportunities for development and ownership of the team. This created high levels of collegiality, creativity and team authority:

> She's got a very collegiate approach and it's her that gels the team really. She taps into what people are good at and draws on those. (*nurse 5*)

Other participants felt that the support and leadership received from their manager was less appropriate, which led to confusion over responsibilities, ownership of the team and its authority. Poor levels of empowerment were demonstrated by one participant and highlighted the need to encourage participation, individual and shared responsibilities and the development of managerial and leadership skills:

> ... I think what would help this team very much is more support from management and our lead clinician. We're very much on our own and a bit more guidance would help: how they want the team to shape; who takes the lead on some things and get things done. It can be muddly sometimes. We get blamed for a lot of things that go wrong. We don't actually get a lot of positive feedback... we never get a well done. (*nurse 6*)

Support within the team

Team working is seen as fundamental to effective practice. Effective teamwork demands a genuine commitment to working together as well as role clarity, solid team working skills and a supportive organisational structure (Hilton, 1995; Ovretveit, 1993; Trnobranski, 1995; Matthias *et al.*, 1997).

Most participants displayed an atmosphere of openness in their team relationships that appeared to lead to candid communication and trust, resulting in effective processes for solving team problems. Recognition of attributes and respect for other members' contributions led to supportive team-working:

> It's a source of great joy to work with other people who you value professionally and respect and who you feel proud to be a part of. (*nurse 8*)

High levels of team support eased feelings of isolation and enabled closer team relationships to be built, although some did not have this experience:

> I think it is a respect thing and sadly nurses are just dreadful to one another... (*nurse 6*)

Concerns were expressed with regard to differing team ideology and whether this would prevent team cohesion and that it would present a non-unified front in the service to the rest of the hospital:

> ... the service is variable. That doesn't have a very good image for us. It's not cohesive. (*nurse 2*)

Personality clashes within the team led to increased stress and team conflict. The benefits of team working are greatly diminished if team members do not confront their differences in a constructive manner (Ovretveit, 1993).

> There's nobody telling us how the team's going to be, so it leaves unrest in the team. I don't think anybody agrees on where we are going.... I think if we had a team leader, it would be better. (*nurse 6*)

Although it was identified that team meetings took place, few identified protected time for team building:

> We have clinical supervision... it's good for clearing the air of bad feelings or feeling you have too much on your plate. It made us close as a team. We were totally reliant on each other for support. (*nurse 5*)

Medical commitment and support

Senior medical commitment and support from the organisation evidently influenced the successful transition of nurses into their new role and the implementation of the service. It was also seen as promoting acceptance of the role and support for the team. Participants experienced different levels of support and commitment from senior medical staff. This, they perceived, was based on whether medical staff believed in outreach, how they felt it would affect their workload, their understanding of the role and how much they valued the team's knowledge and skills:

> ... it's very frustrating because if they won't believe in us, it is very difficult to get everyone else behind you. (*nurse 6*)

Relationships

'Relationships' was the third dominant element to emerge and the constituent clusters included: inter-team collaboration; and communication; and interpersonal skills. Most participants experienced some form of difficulty with relationships that led to varying degrees of anxiety and feelings of isolation. Team support was identified as an essential way of ameliorating these problems. Initiation into the ward environment required highly developed communication skills to build strong relationships.

Inter-team collaboration – ward nursing and medical staff

Participants involved in setting up a service appeared to experience most stress as they were initially viewed with suspicion and hostility by ward nursing and medical staff:

> It made us feel we were treading on eggshells. People would snarl as you went up the ward. It was hideous. (*nurse 8*)

Despite initial difficult relationships, outreach appears to have become an accepted part of ward care, even though problems with junior medical staff have continued. In turn, outreach nurses' opinions of ward staff changed as they came to acknowledge the difficulties that ward staff experience. As ward staff felt less threatened, relationships became more collaborative and participants experienced a sense of belonging:

> We got invited to a Christmas meal on a ward, so that was a definite. (*nurse 1*)

The PRHOs [Pre-Registration House Officers] they look to you for support and guidance. I think it takes a load off them because they have a safety net. (*nurse 3*)

However, outreach team members felt that their standing within the intensive care unit team had altered as they were not perceived as an integral part of the intensive care team. This led to feelings of isolation:

I don't feel part of the ICU team any more. That's a bit of a shock. (*nurse 4*)

Most participants agreed that although the ward staffs' views of intensive care staff had altered considerably since the commencement of outreach, these feelings were not generally reciprocated:

I think it is wrong that they view themselves as elitist... I sometimes think that a good six months on the wards will cure them of that and their high and mighty attitudes. I think it is a lack of realisation of what a good job most ward nurses do when they are faced with such difficulties. (*nurse 8*)

It is interesting to note that despite government directives (Department of Health, 2000a) with regard to 'opening the doors of intensive care units', sharing skills and breaking down barriers, most participants believed that intensive care staff remain firmly behind closed doors.

Communication and interpersonal skills

Initiation into the ward environment required highly developed skills in order to build strong relationships:

You have to be constantly jolly, approachable, helpful, smiling. Nothing's too much trouble. It does wear thin. (*nurse 8*)

Misconceptions about respective roles were evident and often led to barriers, a finding that supports studies on interdisciplinary collaboration.

[From medical staff to outreach team] Who are you? Who do you think you are? A lot of misunderstanding. (*nurse 8*)

At times I would have to stand my ground and argue the point. I hated it. You have to think really hard about going to the registrar because you can alienate those doctors and they won't work with you. (*nurse 2*)

Knowledge and skills

The constituent clusters identified with regard to 'knowledge and skills' were: degree of preparation for the role; decision making; role clarity and accountability; and role development.

Preparation for the role

Individual participants identified varying levels of preparation for the role. Most experienced an induction period from between two to four weeks that they felt was essential and helped to decrease stress levels in the early stages. Some thought that the content was inadequate and therefore felt less competent to undertake the role. The experiences of the first members of individual teams often influenced the content of some programmes and there appeared to be a correlation between leadership style and adequate preparation.

Decision making

The majority of the participants felt that decision making was more complex in the outreach role as they were constantly faced with deteriorating critically ill patients and hospital politics. Decision-making skills improved through experience and team support:

> ... sometimes it's talking about ideas and saying... 'What would you do?' (*nurse 3*)

As the service became more accepted, there was evidence of frequent collaborative working and decision making. Shared learning and acceptance of the service by senior staff were identified as improving team credibility and mutual respect. However, there was evidence of ongoing conflict over junior medical staff decisions which left participants frustrated:

> ... the doctors that don't listen.... You have to walk away. (*nurse 2*)

Role clarity and accountability

Concerns were raised about lack of clarity around role boundaries. This impacted on participants' confidence and made them feel vulnerable:

... because you overstep the role as a nurse you actually put yourself at risk by doing something you shouldn't do. (*nurse 5*)

This underlines recommendations made by Henneman *et al.* (1995) and Coombs and Dillon (2002) which outline the need for role clarification to safeguard patient outcomes.

Role development

The role was seen as an opportunity by all participants to develop new clinical, interpersonal, educational or managerial and leadership skills, and some were undertaking further education for the role. Many felt that the role had given them an insight into the workings of the organisation and the opportunity to build on relationships by networking:

You write guidelines and stuff. You get an appreciation of where the power lies in the hospital. (*nurse 3*)

In turn, some intensive care nurses were concerned that they might lose their specialist skills and felt it important to retain them by working for short periods within intensive care. The study did not reveal that participants with a ward background necessarily felt the same need.

Conclusions and recommendations

The study identified that individuals have a variety of reasons for becoming an outreach team member, but job satisfaction and the opportunity for new challenges and independence appeared to be the biggest motivators.

▨ **Recommendation 1** Managers within critical care need to identify alternative career opportunities in order to retain experienced senior staff within practice.

It is essential that senior management and medical consultants are committed to outreach to ensure its acceptance and continuing success. The study shows that staff members in new roles are continually concerned with practice and accountability issues and the need for sound support systems.

- **Recommendation 2** Organisations should review the management and support structure for critical care outreach nurses to ensure role clarity. Well-designed induction programmes need to be in place to ensure that individuals are prepared for the role.

  It was apparent that effective leadership led to more cohesive working and ownership of the teams which ultimately leads to greater creativity, a common vision, team authority and credibility.

- **Recommendation 3** Review and invest in leadership development for the outreach team.

  Team exposure to ward areas provided a deeper understanding for critical care nurses and helped to break down barriers; in addition, continued support for ward staff led to mutual respect and trust. This enabled a true collaboration of staff working towards a seamless service to improve continuity and quality of patient care.

- **Recommendation 4** Protected team time should be provided to enable team building, professional development and networking to build relationships outside of outreach.

  Critical care outreach services will need to identify the impact they have had on the care of the critically ill ward patient. The future role of outreach services may change as a result, but teams will need to clarify what that role will be, what additional skills and knowledge they require and how this relates to patient care, nursing practice and the NHS of the future.

Part 2
Community stroke services research: a needs-based assessment
Moira Keating

Intention

- To examine service provision for people who have experienced stroke
- To explore user perception of current service provision

Introduction

Every year in England and Wales about 100,000 people have their first stroke, and the disabilities can be severe and long-lasting (The Stroke Association, 1997). The cost of long-term care is estimated at 5.8% of the National Health Service's and social services' expenditure. These costs are based on long-term outlay and increasing prevalence (The Stroke Association, 1998).

Each year one semi-rural town in the east of England is estimated to have 313 new stroke cases and 938 survivors living in the community, 469 of whom will have a significant disability, and 75% will have been admitted to hospital during the acute phase (North Essex Health Authority, 2000). The long-term benefits of secondary care are lost without good community support and liaison when the patient leaves hospital; efficient discharge planning and community rehabilitation are therefore essential (Pollock, 1997; North Essex Health Authority, 2000). Recovery from stroke can continue over a long time and rehabilitation should continue until maximum recovery has been achieved; some patients require ongoing support for many years (Department of Health, 2001b).

The NHS Plan (Department of Health, 2000a) has set out the Government's programme of investment and reform, and *Modernising Social Services* (Department of Health, 1998) puts forward the Government's proposals to improve social services, promote independence and raise standards. The *National Service Framework (NSF) for Older People* (Department of Health, 2001b) outlines the Government's targets for delivering improved health and social care to older people; it aims to promote standards of care, extend access to services, ensure fairer funding, develop services that promote independence and help older people stay healthy.

Standard 5 of the *NSF for Older People* relates to stroke and is aimed at all ages. It focuses on prevention, immediate care, early and continuing rehabilitation and long-term support. Stroke is considered a long-term condition. The need to improve the management of long-term conditions within the health service is a significant challenge for the NHS and as a response the Government has published an NHS and social care model to support local innovation and integration (Department of Health, 2005). Wilkinson and Murray (1998) comment that, historically, much service provision has been service- rather than needs-led and has been offered at the convenience of the provider rather than the patient. All the Government documents convey the premise that the needs of patients are now central to the philosophy of the NHS, and the fact that patients may have different ideas about the effects of their health on, for example, employment or transport availability.

This needs-based assessment (NA) investigated the 'need' requirement and long-term psychosocial support available within a county borough. The project was jointly funded by a Healthcare Trust and County Council social services,

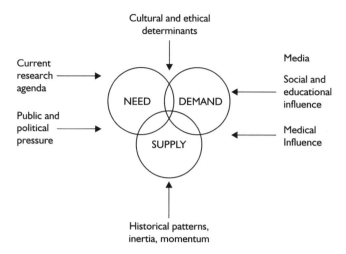

Figure 5.1 Need, demand and supply: influences and overlaps (Stevens and Raftery, 1994).

with the support of the community voluntary service, The Stroke Association (TSA) and the local advocacy scheme.

There are a number of different approaches to NA, e.g. comparative, corporate and epidemiological. This NA used a corporate approach, which is based on the demands, wishes and alternative perspectives of interested parties, giving insight and detail on local discrepancies of need, supply and demand (Stevens and Raftery, 1994; Stevens and Bickler, 2000). Need is defined as the 'population's ability to benefit from health care'. Benefit is interpreted comprehensively to include general wellbeing and benefit for third parties. Whilst need is ideally kept distinct from the assessment of demand and supply, the three overlap (van den Bos and Triemstra, 1999; Rawaf and Orton, 2000; Stevens and Bickler, 2000). Figure 5.1 depicts how needs, demand and supply may overlap and differ.

Background

The project arose following the need to relocate a small voluntary-run speech and language group that had met within a health care rehabilitation facility; relocation was necessary because of building closure. As the stroke coordinator for the north of an eastern county I convened a cross-service multi-disciplinary team that included NHS, social services, and voluntary service professionals and the Speech and Language group's representative, to consider both the relocation and expansion of the voluntary dysphasia group's services. This gathering of professionals argued that the local services to stroke patients were poorly tailored to requirements; however, there was little local evidence to support or reject this hypothesis. It was therefore felt that a formal research project was required for which the group set aims and objectives.

This research is a corporate NA of the services and support available to people with stroke sequela after discharge from inpatient rehabilitation in the local borough. The aim was to identify priorities in service provision in order to benefit stroke individuals and the wider stroke population. Although there has been success in reducing the mortality rates for stroke this has automatically increased the burden of chronic disease (The Stroke Association, 1998; Office for National Statistics, 1997; Martin *et al.*, 1988). Chronically ill patients are particularly likely to benefit from NA and the routine use of patient-derived data in making decisions about the distribution, access and content of long-term care (van den Bos and Triemstra, 1999).

It is anticipated that this research will help inform local commissioners and service providers about local services, as well as client and professional opinions, and thereby facilitate appropriate action to meet governmental locally.

The study

The aims of this project were to:

- Identify from the literature what interventions enable people who have experienced a stroke, and have completed their rehabilitation, to maintain or improve their quality of life and reintegrate into social and/or occupational activities.
- Identify what types of service presently exist for this group within the community and what these services presently provide, to whom and by whom.
- Identify what the post-stroke population and service providers think of the present provision and what service they feel they need that will maintain or improve their quality of life and reintegration into the mainstream community.
- Analyse data in relation to present service provision and compare them with what is viewed by the literature as being effective, the aim being to identify areas of conformity and dissonance.
- Recommend service development/changes from conclusions of this research.

The methodology for the study used a combination of both quantitative and qualitative data collection and analysis to provide a measurable and in-depth study (Cormack, 1996). A survey research design, using postal questionnaires to service providers and a separate simultaneous questionnaire for service users, was selected to collect data about practice and provision of services to stroke survivors (Hastings, 1996). The service providers survey was sent to 250 services and there was a 32% return rate. The service user survey went to 50 clients and there was a 50% return rate. This approach provided the most practical and cost-effective means of gathering data (Judd *et al.*, 1991). Further qualitative data from focus groups were gathered to understand the thoughts and perceptions of service provider and users (Roberts, 1997; Reed and Roskell-Payton, 1997).

This study cannot be considered a comprehensive record of services available to people following stroke in the local borough. In addition, the method of questionnaire distribution, which was only established on one database, and a low questionnaire response rate of 32%, means that the results of the study have limited generalisation. Therefore the results must be evaluated with the understanding that this investigation provides us with an unfinished picture of how and what services are made available and accessed by clients following stroke in this area.

The client survey received a disappointing response. However, every effort had been made to obtain a representative sample of clients following stroke. Previous surveys of similar clients by the Acute Trust also produced poor response rates. It is reasoned that the disabilities of this group of clients reduce the possibility of them being motivated or able to reply to such survey requests.

The findings

The findings from client questionnaires indicate that groups and services are used, but not all clients find that their needs are met, particularly in terms of informational and emotional requirements. This is of concern, as previous research has identified three types of social support – informational, emotional and instrumental – as being significantly related to recovery of functional capacity (Glass and Maddox, 1992; Swartzman *et al.*, 1998) (Figure 5.2).

However, paradoxically, according to the provider questionnaire, groups and organisations often provided information and emotional support (Figure 5.3).

The social context of the clients' needs was also emphasised. It was identified from both the focus group data and questionnaires that there is a lack of understanding of the patients' view point and that professionals have limited understanding of clients' needs. The issues identified by the provider focus group are group into three themes: 'realistic', 'knowledge' and 'remodelling'.

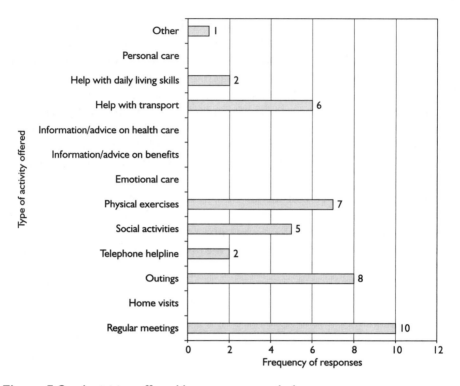

Figure 5.2 Activities offered by groups attended.

The providers considered needs by deliberating on how 'need' was currently driven and also pragmatically in terms of economic resources. The general feeling was that as services and individual professionals they did not really look truthfully at what client/patient and carer needs really were:

That is the big issue at the moment we go in and treat for this, then this.

If they start walking then we can move away.

Society was seen to exclude those with disabilities, and acts of law do not automatically rectify this omission. The promotion of client/patient dignity and choice was also expressed and was linked with the call for a client/patient needs-led service:

Just being accepted as human beings and not talked down to.

Agreement on the inadequacy and inertia of current services was comprehensive in all areas of service provision to stroke patients/clients:

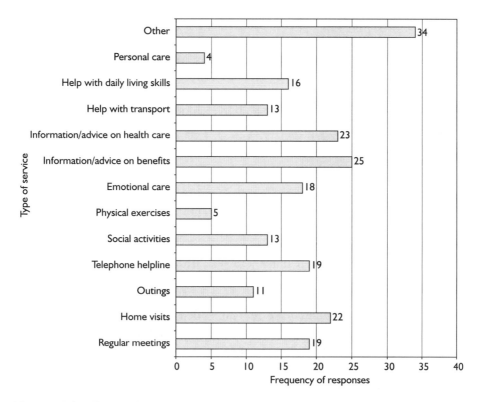

Figure 5.3 Types of service provided.

So we just feel that everything is spread very thin but there are people out there working their socks off.

However, the belief that creativity and innovation in the way in which future care provision is provided was seen as central to developing a client/patient needs-led service:

... we start engaging with those services organisations and groups that are out there that we can use in a different way maybe.

The main themes of the client focus groups were 'understanding' and 'self'.

The overwhelming desire by the clients was for understanding. This theme imbued all the discussion, whether understanding for themselves, the professionals who cared for them, or the general public. There were strong expressions of a desire to have a complete understanding of what happened to them and how it has rendered parts of themselves dysfunctional, and continues to affect them on a daily basis:

When I got home, like the emotional side, I wasn't told.

Diverse support needs were expressed, along with the need for development, encouragement and practical backup, in addition to the informational needs already discussed. Emotional needs were diverse and were felt to be completely unrecognised and wholly unmet for both the patient and carers:

They want everyone out of hospital and getting better at home and then nobody helps.

There are problems relating to service provision, bureaucratic barriers and poor communication between primary and secondary care. In addition, there is limited support at home to enable clients to develop coping skills and become less isolated, as well as recognition of the need for social recovery. This research also identified that there was little opportunity to talk about changes of identity and self and a reduction of life's previously normal activities.

Earlier subjective studies have recommended the need to improve social support and post-stroke clients' quality of life (Pound and Gompertz, 1998; Burton, 2000). Consequently, there is a need to extend access to services, ensure fairer funding and develop services that promote independence. These would meet government targets and concur with other research findings (King, 1996; Department of Health, 1998, 2001b; Kim *et al.*, 1999; Williams *et al.*, 1999; Carod-Artal *et al.*, 2000).

There is anecdotal evidence that local professionals have argued for increased prominence of stroke support groups to provide social support and information to stroke survivors. Research verifies this professional view and that stroke support groups have a high level of knowledge about stroke and stroke prevention (van Veenendaal *et al.*, 1996; Welterman *et al.*, 2000). This relates to the notion of the expert patient. The provider focus group confirmed that professionals advocate stroke support groups and the client questionnaire data confirmed that 52% of survey respondents attended or contemplated attending local stroke support groups.

Survey information showed that support groups provide a broad range of services that increase social activities for clients (see Figures 5.2 and 5.3), a point confirmed by previous research (Geddes and Chamberlain, 1994; Oehring and Oakley, 1994). However, the client focus group did not discuss stroke groups as an area of information or support. The study by van Veenendaal *et al.* (1996) also found that stroke survivors did not call for stroke groups to be more prominent as providers of information. Therefore, although informational support appears to be available it is either inappropriate or is not currently accessed adequately.

Recommendations

This research has identified areas of support that would benefit stroke survivors from the onset of stroke and within the community. How this support is provided requires negotiation and discussion locally between the current provider and service commissioners. Therefore these recommendations will provide principles for innovative changes in care to be made:

- A structured educational programme should be implemented for each person, based on each person's diagnosis and individual needs at onset of stroke, continuing through into the long term, the documentation of which is held by the client.
- Development of strategies that will reduce existing boundaries of service, especially those caused by age, diagnosis and funding-related inequalities.
- The encouragement of pioneering strategies to integrate voluntary and statutory sector services to meet client needs imaginatively.
- Voluntary and statutory sector services should be developed, with a special focus on training and advancing nursing staff skills to enhance clients' acquisition of coping skill and personal independence.
- The introduction of a specialist counselling service to meet the emotional challenges that stroke survivors and their carers/families encounter during the recovery from stroke.
- A comprehensive information system should be developed that uses conventional advertising and computer technology and the Internet. Access to a wide range of information about strokes should be provided on a local web site and other endorsed web sites and there should be areas for providers to advertise their services.

Implications

It is now widely recognised that modernising health and social services is essential and is an area that is governmentally led by *The NHS Plan* (Department of Health, 2000b), *Modernising Social Services* (Department of Health, 1998), the *NSF for Older People* (Department of Health, 2001b) and *Supporting People with Long Term Conditions* (Department of Health, 2005). These papers outline areas of investment and reform, and are aimed at extending access to services, ensuring fairer funding, and developing services that promote independence and support local innovation and integration within voluntary and statutory sector services. These are all areas that have been acknowledged in this research as issues affecting patients and the recommendations are based around implementing ideas that will realise these directives to ensure a more client-led service.

The study gives informed details on local discrepancies of need, supply and demand, and enlightens local commissioners and service providers about local services and client and professional opinions. Enabling appropriate action required meeting the objectives of the government papers locally. The recommendations are focused on ensuring patients' needs, as identified by this research and the literature, and are met by the local services ensuring a more client-led service. If these proposals are not put into operation services will continue to be service led and will not meet those needs perceived as important by clients and local service providers. This could potentially mean that the use of the funds for stroke care locally is inefficient.

The cost of caring for patients following stroke for the health and social care sectors is estimated to be 5.8% of their budgets (The Stroke Association, 1998). Funding allocation will continue to be inequitable for stroke services if bureaucratic barriers and poor communication continues between service sectors.

Conclusion

This Need Assessment (NA) has been a partnership between the health, social and voluntary sectors. Collaborative working has major benefits, even though it is more difficult to organise than single agency working. Wilkinson and Murray (1998) point out that many health needs cannot be met by health services alone. Cultural changes in the NHS that have occurred since the publication of the white papers *The New NHS: Modern, Dependable* (Department of Health, 1997) and *Saving Lives: Our Healthier Nation* (Department of Health, 1999) raise issues about assessment. The emphasis is now on the wider determinants of health and decreasing health inequalities, and the culture has changed from one of competition to collaboration. NA requires the involvement of services from the voluntary sector and local authorities, as well as all NHS organisations.

Voluntary and local authority organisations provide many activities that are not specifically for stroke survivors; however, they do have a positive effect on health. This has to be viewed as extending and increasing the types of intervention available within a community, and it therefore increases the number of organisations involved in NA. It is heartening that in this NA there was enthusiasm from all sector services to change practice and a recognition that clients' needs are not, at the time of research, central to their service.

The NA had many ethical challenges: expert relationships in working together and mutual problem-solving skills were crucial. Developing close operational relationships with key individuals who are employees/volunteers within each organisation was essential to enable completion of the survey distribution in particular.

Developing relationships with the 'doers' in partnership organisations is essential. However, in practice, when working with voluntary organisations this is not always straightforward, as volunteers are unpaid helpers and there is a reliance on their willingness to take part. It can be surprising and challenging to find out who are the 'movers and shakers' within organisations. The research required a broader understanding of who had authority and needed a more political and diplomatic approach to the partnerships involved, particularly when disseminating the final report and recommendations.

The project was rewarding and the partnerships made continue to be helpful and supportive in working in the local stroke service.

Part 3
Initial assessments in community specialist palliative care: an evaluation of nurses' perceptions and experiences
Rachel Wilson

Intention

- To examine delivery of community palliative specialist care services in a locality
- To examine the impact of community palliative specialist care assessment on interpersonal relations

Introduction

The initial assessment of a patient's specialist palliative care needs is vital in ensuring that the most appropriate resources are used in the ongoing management and care of the patient. If this initial assessment is not accurate then it not only has financial implications for the hospice, but also patients may not receive what is appropriate for their needs. The National Institute for Clinical Excellence (NICE) (2004) concurs that inadequate assessment of patients' physical symptoms and psychosocial needs leads to 'failure to recognise their needs for supportive and palliative care, resulting in necessary services being denied to them'. Effective assessment hinges on the 'provision of appropriate education and training for health and social care professionals, feasible and sensitive assessment tools and the availability of skilled personnel' (NICE, 2004).

The hospice setting for this research study takes the view that interdisciplinary assessments are the 'ideal' model of assessment, because of the different perspectives that can be brought to an assessment. It is inevitable, however, that limited staff resources mean that most of the time the nurse will carry out the assessment alone. How do nurses actually feel about these single assessments? Do they feel pressurised to produce a 'perfect' holistic assessment on their own? What happens in the interactions between the nurses and others? What support do they get and what were the expectations? What can be learnt from their experiences?

Background

In the past, patients tended to be referred for specialist palliative care only when they were in the terminal phase of their illness. Increasingly, however, it is being seen as an integral part of care, and is often delivered alongside cancer treatment services. The Department of Health therefore commissioned NICE to develop evidence-based and specialist palliative care guidance, which was published in March 2004. The aim of the guidance is to ensure that patients and carers receive high-quality information, communication, symptom control, and psychological, social and spiritual support at key points in their cancer journey: namely, at diagnosis, commencement and completion of treatment, disease recurrence, when disease becomes incurable, when dying is diagnosed and any time at the patient's request.

Assessment

The World Health Organization (1987) described assessment as consisting of 'receiving and gathering data about the needs of persons for nursing care'. The Cancer Research Campaign (1993) defined the purpose of the assessment interview as 'to determine the exact nature and extent of a patient's problems, his or her reactions to them and the nature and impact of treatment'. NICE (2004) concurs that the assessment is a crucial first step in ensuring that patients' needs are identified and goes further in recognising that the process should 'fully reflect the shared nature of assessment between patients and professionals and should support patients in assessing their own needs'. This historical process demonstrates a progression from a technically accurate yet somewhat unfeeling definition of a one-way process of assessing, through to the shared nature of assessment between patients and professionals, supporting patients to assess their own needs and thus creating a partnership.

The study

A qualitative design was used for this research in order to explore the perceptions and experiences of community specialist palliative care nurses undertaking initial assessments of patients and families facing a life-threatening illness. This study was an attempt to gain insight into the nurses' thoughts and feelings and the meanings attributed to them. Therefore, a phenomenological philosophy was thought to be an appropriate framework to guide thinking about the research design. Phenomenology is part of the humanistic tradition and is a philosophy that seeks to make sense of reality and emphasises the uniqueness of human beings. The foundations of phenomenology were developed by Husserl and elaborated on by others, including Schutz and Heidegger (Bernard, 2000). The research design was also influenced by the grounded theory approach (Glaser and Strauss, 1967).

The sample group comprised five nurses who were community Macmillan nurses, with more than three years' specialist palliative care experience. The sample size of five is relatively small; however, no new information was received, which indicated data saturation and that comparisons between variables were not being considered.

Unstructured interview was the technique used to collect the data. Unstructured interviews are really guided conversations or 'conversations with a purpose' (Burgess, 1984). They are very versatile and are excellent in building rapport between interviewer and interviewee. The interviews provided a depth and richness to the study, giving a unique insight into the live experiences of the assessment process by the nurses.

Findings

An examination for commonalities among the participants' beliefs generated five discreet themes: conflict; cognitive processes; human responses; power and control; and role. The relationship between and among these themes was then explored and it became apparent that there was a socio-psychological 'dance' that the participants experienced when meeting a patient for the first time. This involved experiencing the five themes, both interpersonally and intra-personally, as the participants sought to make sense of them, so that they could achieve the best possible outcome for the patient, carers and themselves. This 'strategic manoeuvring' became ever-present and was apparent from the point of the participant receiving the referral form, into the assessment and beyond.

The key to grounded theory is that the researcher must discover the core category that links all other themes and which is the basic social-psychological process involved in the research. This was identified as 'strategic manoeuvres' and was the phenomenon that was most significant to the participants in this research study. 'Strategic manoeuvres' demonstrates the intrapersonal (internal) and interpersonal (external) dynamics of the five discreet themes of conflict, cognitive processes, human responses, power and control and role that the participants experienced when performing a specialist palliative care assessment.

The term 'strategic manoeuvres', was derived from Goffman's (1970) work on strategic interaction that explained the socio-psychological 'games' that people employed when relating to each other. He described them as (1) 'face-games', where each participant 'manoeuvres' to maximise his or her valued identity whilst seeking an equilibrium to enable others to do the same; (2) 'relationship-games', where the participants seek to create, maintain or terminate relationships; (3) 'exploitation-games', where the participants seek to maximise their position of power over one another; and (4) 'information-games', where the participants seek to conceal as well as uncover certain kinds of knowledge. Goffman's (1970) work perfectly reflects the core category and the basic socio-psychological process of 'strategic manoeuvres' found in this study.

The findings provide a unique perspective on the experiences of five community specialist palliative care nurses who undertake assessments of patients in their homes. The subjective phenomenology of their experiences cannot be questioned, but how did the literature support the findings of this research and what has been learnt?

The most relevant piece of work that related to the first meeting between the nurse and the patient was not a nursing paper, but one written by Laungani (2002), who is a counsellor. The paper examined the nature of the first interview between the counsellor and the client, when both are attempting to form their impressions of one another. The participants concurred with Laungani (2002) in that the concept of 'first impressions' was vital in building an effective trusting relationship to enable ongoing meaningful work to take place; therefore, all other findings in the research need to be considered in relation to this concept.

Laungani's (2002) paper discussed three major problems that arise in the process of forming first impressions. These are maintaining neutrality and objectivity, exercising cognitive control, and expressing empathy. The paper describes the first interview as a game with its own set of rules, where some of the rules are covert and remain unknown to the client, placing the client at a certain disadvantage. The first interview is crucial in that it sets the scene and creates a template for future work. The client and counsellor (nurse and patient) are each making a judgement or an assessment of each other. Palliative care patients may consider the counsellor or nurse to be an expert who will solve all their problems, or to possessing 'magico-spiritual' powers; in other words, as a 'god-like' figure who holds all the answers to questions of life and death.

Conflict

The literature reviewed demonstrated that 'conflict' was mainly experienced in relation to the intrapersonal and interpersonal ethical considerations. This concurred with the participants, as they spoke of conflict in terms of feeling pressurised to collude with family members by hiding from them the facts of the patient's illness. The conflict for the participants was that they must consider the ethical implications, in that the patient has a right to know his or her disease state and prognosis. The discussion surrounding ethical considerations was based on 'determining the right thing to do' (Megel and Elrod, 1993) and balancing conflict in relation to not only their avoidance of collusion, but also the patient's understanding of his or her disease state and the participant's sense of what the patient wants to know. This linked in with the human responses and power and control themes as the participants sought to maintain control in a precarious situation:

> I don't wish to actively collude with anybody, um, and I find it really hard in those situations where perhaps the family meet you on the door-step and say 'well granny doesn't know the whole implications of it, and not to tell her, OK', um, that I find very difficult but I always say to the family that if she asks me a direct question I can't lie to her, it wouldn't be fair, and I won't lie to her, if she doesn't ask me the direct question, I'm not going to fire it in to see what's going on... it's about trying to establish some boundary...' (*Interviewee 4*)

As well as ethical conflicts, other interpersonal conflicts identified by the participants were related to working relationships, particularly with district nurses, general practitioners and other disciplines within the hospice. Whilst this finding agreed with some of the literature, particularly the work of Megel and Elrod (1993), Wright (2001) and Skilbeck and Seymour (2002), there is no supportive work relating to conflict around interdisciplinary specialist palliative care assessments. The literature cited above discussed role conflict, but only in relation to colleagues' perceptions. The participants in this study felt conflict around not only colleagues' perceptions but also the patients' and carers' perceptions of their role.

Conflict is not necessarily a negative concept, and the literature has even suggested that it can be a catalyst for change; however, serious interpersonal conflicts that are poorly managed have adverse effects upon relationship functioning (Megel and Elrod, 1993). Understanding the point of view and needs of others, as well as maintaining relationships whilst protecting others from hurt within the conflict, is characteristic of the 'caring perspective' (Megel and Elrod, 1993); the participants in this study demonstrated this 'caring perspective' and the consequential conflict they experienced. Little seems to be known about the effects of intrapersonal conflict, but the participants in this study highlighted time pressures, tiredness and stress as factors as adding to their conflict in an assessment session.

Cognitive processes

Cognitive processes were clearly an important part of the participants' 'strategic manoeuvres' when balancing thought processes with the other themes. The literature supported the findings, particularly Barker (1997) who described the 'interview as a conversation' with the aim of relationship building, collaboration, problem identification and problem solving. These are all aspects of the cognitive processes identified by the participants. The unique finding from this current study was the participants' 'pre-assessment' of the forthcoming meeting with the patient and carers. This was based on what was written on the referral form, the referrer being the patient, family member, friend, nurse, social worker or doctor:

> You know sometimes you get, perhaps, expecting you to come with 'Well I've been told you do everything', create miracles, that sort of stuff, or, um, or, there may be those who feel that you're going to keep coming, so I think maybe for me that's, sort of, the start of the assessment is where people are on the phone. (*Interviewee 5*)

This links in with the concept of 'first impressions' and is key in getting the 'conversation' off to a good start, setting the scene and creating a template for future work (Barker, 1997; Laungani, 2002).

First impressions are an intrapersonal dynamic, but involve all five of the themes in this study. The participants in this study expressed a view that if another professional assessed a patient on their behalf, then this affected their ongoing work, somehow losing the intimacy of the relationship. This study has not ascertained patients' views; however, the literature concurs with the participants' views on first impressions in that it is the crucial first step in forming relationships:

> I think it is, it is the visit when you really set terms, I think it is one of the most crucial, any first visit, any first introductions to any part of the service are fundamentally important to get it right as you can, but it's so important, not to blunder in there, be insensitive in any way, but just to be guided by the individual in the house, um, their space and not to delve into things that they're not comfortable with. (*Interviewee 3*)

Laungani's (2002) paper describes 'cognitive control' as an element of the counsellor putting on a 'professional face' when meeting a client. It allows the counsellor to exercise some degree of control over the interview, by remaining calm in the face of emotional outbursts by the client. This has parallels with the cognitive processes, power and control, and role themes in the current study. The participants sought to make sense of what they saw and heard in order to help the patient and carers, both physically and psychosocially, whilst at the same time attempting to stay in control in an uncertain situation.

Laungani (2002) states that the counsellor, as well as the client, is actively involved in forming first impressions. Despite the participants' assertions that they go into a first meeting with a patient with a 'blank sheet' or 'empty page', the suggestion is made that this neutrality and objectivity is impossible. According to Laungani (2002), positive and negative first impressions create their own positive and negative 'halo' effects. For example, if a community specialist palliative care nurse is judged favourably by the patient, then he or she will be seen in positive terms, despite objective evidence to the contrary that he or she represents the hospice and death.

The participants struggled to explain how they structured an assessment session. That is not to say that they did not have a framework, but verbalising what they did seemed difficult. They appeared to rely on the hospice's interdisciplinary notes as a guideline to assess patients' physical, psychosocial and spiritual needs. Doctors have a clear structure to their assessments; however, this assessment is based around physical symptoms, family and social history in relation to illness (Toghill, 1994), which is different from the participants' holistic assessment of the physical, psychosocial and spiritual aspects of a person. The medical assessment is a cognitive process and is described in the medical field as 'clinical reasoning' that is based around diagnosing medical problems using decision-making and problem-solving skills (Round, 2001).

Barker's (1997) opinion on mental health assessments is that 'structure provides security' and a structured interview is likely to provoke less anxiety for both the nurse and patient. However, the findings show that the participants' assessments are based on what confronts them in the first meeting. Barker asserts that a flexible framework comes with experience, which is what the participants believed. However, he states that this flexibility must be within a firm structure and this structure is something the participants were unable to describe. All this relates to the themes of human responses and cognitive processes in the current research, where the participants strove to make the assessment as patient-centred as possible whilst ensuring that critical information for decision making was gathered.

Human responses

Human responses were identified as having intrapersonal dynamics, but with a direct impact on interpersonal dynamics. The literature supports the participants' experiences of the importance of relationship building by establishing trust, honesty and rapport from the first meeting, and by demonstrating warmth, empathy, congruence and unconditional positive regard (Barker, 1997; Cutcliffe *et al.*, 2001; Laungani, 2002):

> I work towards being very honest with people and try to get that over to people fairly early on, you know, there's nothing that you can ask me that will bother me, you know, you've got to be honest, for them to trust... (*Interviewee 2*)

> ... I mean obviously there's inevitably there's information gathering but I think it's about relationship, it's about, I think, I don't know 'cos I've never been on the receiving side of that, but I can guess, if I felt that someone was taking some time and taking some interest in everything else I would feel much more empathy towards that person than more than just, you know, that wanting just to do a tick sheet of this, this, this and this... and I think that for me would make a difference with ongoing working with that person... (*Interviewee 1*)

How this relationship was forged depended on a number of factors, including time, but mainly the relationship was affected adversely if the community specialist palliative care nurse, who was to carry on working with the patient, did not perform that first assessment. This did not necessarily imply that an assessment by another professional was not accurate, but the participants felt that some intimacy was missing from the ongoing relationship with the patient. This 'relationship' between the participant and the patient and the development of empathic understanding is closely aligned to a counsellor's relationship with a client; it would be unlikely that counsellors would have someone else assess on his or her behalf, even in an interdisciplinary context.

The first meeting creates fear and uncertainty for both the patient and participant, a finding that is supported by Laungani (2002). The participants in this study were acutely aware of the patients' abilities to form their own first impressions, particularly around attributing the nurse with 'god-like' qualities and representing death, resulting in a 'pre-assessment' by the nurses before meeting the patient which involved both cognitive and emotional responses:

> ... it can be daunting walking into a complete unknown, um, scene, you don't know what you're going to find out, maybe someone in a lot of pain, maybe someone very angry, very distressed, um, so a lot of uncertainty... (*Interviewee 5*)

There was an abundance of literature that addressed the patient's fear and uncertainty (Edwards and Miller, 2001; Heaven and Maguire, 1998); however, there was little to parallel the participants' expressions of their fear of the unknown. Therefore it may be important for further work to be carried out around the fear experienced by the community specialist palliative care nurse when anticipating an assessment.

Specialist palliative care nurses are increasingly engaged in emotional and therapeutic interventions with patients and their families (Cancer Relief Macmillan Fund, 1995) and this is reflected in the human responses theme in this current study. Supervision is a process that can provide a means for the nurses to assimilate and make sense of complex feelings, whilst at the same time using them as a guide to understanding the feelings of patients (Jones, 1999).

Power and control

Power and control was an important theme in the 'strategic manoeuvres' encountered by the participants in balancing the interpersonal and intrapersonal dynamics. As stated above, Laungani's (2002) paper describes the first interview as being like a game with its own set of rules, where some of the rules are covert and remain unknown to the client. This could be likened to the participants having knowledge about a patient before meeting them, creating an imbalance of power.

The participants in this study described the delicate balance they experience when deciding whether or not to give bad news to a patient. James and Field's (1996) paper discusses the patients' rights to information and the participants concur with this view; however, they felt that an important part of their role was to be 'gatekeepers' of information. Their intention was not to cause harm by giving 'bad news' to a patient who was not ready to hear it, but it was not clear from this study how the participants came to that conclusion, other than under-standing patients through building trust and rapport:

> I will always say I've got limited information so it's no good asking me what's happening on the first visit... first of all are they the sort of person that wants to know? Because it's Pandora's Box, if you ask me, and I know and I tell you, you can't take the information back, and we all ask because we want the good answer... *(Interviewee 4)*

Caution must therefore be taken when making this decision on behalf of the patient. Page (1999) concurs that the effect of power, control and influence by a professional over another is something of which the professional may be unaware. Effective supervision is crucial in raising the self-awareness of nurses who work uni-professionally in order for this potential power imbalance to be identified, maintaining the safety of both nurse and patient.

The participants in this study described their experiences of feeling out of control in assessment situations. Establishing relationship boundaries was a way for them to bring clarity and control to an uncertain situation and this linked closely to the sub-category of collusion in the conflict theme, as dis-cussed earlier. There was a need for the participants to assess the patients with whom they were going to have an ongoing relationship, because if someone else assessed the patient, for whatever reason, then this affected the intimacy of the relationship. This has already been discussed in relation to building rapport in the human responses theme, but it could equally be viewed as the participants feeling a sense of powerlessness and needing to be in control:

> ... if I know that I've been away on holiday, and I've not done a first assessment, it's never quite the same, you don't seem to have that thing which registers in my brain so I guess that that for me is an important, and that's very important to get their sense of what's going on... *(Inter-viewee 2)*

Role

The antithesis of being in control is empowering and enabling, which was something the participants identified as an important part of their role. This concurs with the views of Barker (1997), Wright (2001), Skilbeck and Seymour (2002) and the Royal College of Nursing (2003). Much has been written about the 'role' of the nurse, although there is little information about specialist pal-liative care nurses' role in relation to assessments. The participants identified experience, knowledge and intuition as important aspects of their role, a view supported by the literature; however, they also experienced conflict in relation to others' perceptions of their role. This role conflict centred on patients' poor understanding of their role as well as colleagues' lack of acknowledgment of their work:

> I think sometimes the idea of being a Macmillan nurse is that you're, you know, second to God and knowing a bit about everything and that just isn't so... (*Interviewee 1*)

Barker (1997) asserts that the nurse must demonstrate warmth, empathy, genuineness and unconditional positive regard towards the patient. This supports the participants' perception that their role is not just about 'doing for' but 'being with' the patient, a view that is also supported by Cutcliffe *et al.* (2001) when comparing and contrasting mental health nursing with palliative care nursing.

> I believe in this sort of self and I think a lot of what nurses do with people is, the nurse as a therapist, and I think what that means to people, well, it's very difficult, I think it's actually difficult to define and for me it's the being with people, in terms it sounds sort of corny in some ways, people underestimate what they can offer people, and just the skills that are there, and they're really amazed by the time perhaps they've spent a few years in nursing, but it means an awful lot to a family who are in distress or whatever and that can be just as much a therapy as knowing what their symptoms are... (*Interviewee 3*)

Conclusion and recommendations

Assessments in nursing are the first crucial step in the nursing process. Assessing involves the use of developed skills of observing, communicating, analysing and interpreting; however, although the shared nature of assessments between patients and professionals is acknowledged in the literature, there seems to be little evidence to demonstrate how this is to be achieved.

The findings of this research study have demonstrated that an assessment of a patient requiring specialist palliative care is a more complex process than is suggested by the current literature on nurse assessment. They also showed that community specialist palliative care nurses require a high degree of cognitive skills for problem solving and symptom control, as well as having an understanding of psychosocial issues, whilst demonstrating empathy and forming a trusting, therapeutic relationship with the patient requiring specialist palliative care.

The NHS Cancer Plan (Department of Health, 2000c) identifies key objectives in developing palliative care. These include improving access to care, enhancing the continuity of care and paying attention to patients' experiences of care. Whilst it is essential to listen to and act on patients' experiences, unless the specialist palliative care nurses' experiences are paid equal attention, then it could be argued that the 'shared' experience will be meaningless. In order to bring together both patient and nurse experiences, wider research should be carried out on the concept of first impressions, from both the patients' and nurses' perspectives, given the importance of these in relationship building in the field of specialist palliative care.

- **Recommendation 1** This study has highlighted the importance of first impressions in an assessment and therefore it is recommended that heightening this awareness amongst all specialist palliative care workers through education is essential in improving the experience of patients.
- **Recommendation 2** This study has demonstrated that it is important for community specialist palliative care nurses to perform first assessments in order to maintain intimacy and for a trusting relationship to develop. In order for this to happen, it is recommended that sufficient human and financial resources in the workplace should be made available.
- **Recommendation 3** In order to practice at a level expected of specialist palliative care nurses, the participants have, in this research, identified experience and intuition as vital components of their role in an assessment. I therefore concur with Kratz (1979) and recommend that the most experienced nurses should directly undertake assessments for the benefit of the patients, whilst observing and teaching less experienced nurses.
- **Recommendation 4** The participants in this study were unclear as to how they structured a specialist palliative care assessment session, perhaps implying that they have never been formally taught the art. They relied very much on experience and intuition, which UK nurses identify as important aspects of their practice (Royal College of Nursing, 2003); however, it is recommended that more education on how to structure an assessment session in specialist palliative care is provided, utilising the approaches from the medical, mental health and counselling services. This would ensure a more uniform and holistic approach to specialist palliative care nurse assessments, whilst giving more breadth and depth to it, as well as reducing anxiety for both patient and nurse.
- **Recommendation 5** Specialist palliative care nurse assessment involves intrapersonal and interpersonal 'strategic manoeuvres' relating to conflict, cognitive processes, human responses, power and control, and role on the part of the nurse, and is probably mirrored by the patient and carers. It is recommended, therefore, that these findings could be used as a tool for supervisors to guide and facilitate specialist palliative care nurses in their complex work with patients and families.

Unless the complex process of holistic assessment is addressed in the education and supervision of nurses from student to specialist, then the art and science of nurse assessment may well be lost to the detriment of patient care.

Part 4
Common partnership themes
Kimmy Eldridge

Introduction

All three studies were motivated by the desire to improve the future planning of services. Carpenter's Acute Trust has yet to develop a critical care outreach team as outlined by the Department of Health (Department of Health, 2000a). The study was undertaken to learn from the experience of nurses working in critical outreach as a basis to plan a future local critical care outreach initiative. Keating identified that local services were not being tailored to meet the needs of stroke patients. The aim of the study was to identify the perspectives/ wishes of stakeholders in order to set service priorities that benefit patients. Wilson's study originated from the observation that the hospice's 'ideal' model of interdisciplinary assessment was not consistently being practised because of resource constraints. Wilson is a senior manager of the hospice who observed that, although the hospice community nurses worked within an interdisciplinary context, they were mainly performing assessments alone.

None of the studies' objectives suggest partnership working as an explicit intention. Nonetheless, they illustrate a partnership approach to service planning, a departure from the traditional, hierarchical and adversarial relationships between managers and the managed (Tomlinson, 2005).

The research design and recommendations

All three papers employ a qualitative research design that is appropriate to the research questions. Interview was the chosen data-collection tool for the first two studies, while the third used focus groups to elicit the views of participants. Embedded in these approaches is the philosophical principle that the views and experiences of the participants are legitimate and of value (Gubrium and Holstein, 2002), a philosophy that concords with partnership working (Freeth, 2001).

Keating also employed a postal questionnaire that was distributed to all service providers and users. The survey aimed to establish the level of service provided at the time of the research. Keating conceded that this was the most practical and cost-effective means of gathering data. While this argument may be acceptable for the population at large, it raises the question of appropriateness in the context of this particular client group. Using this tool to assess health needs also raises a further moral issue: is it ethical to employ an assessment tool if it is not accessible to the target audience? Keating found that the users' response to the questionnaire was 'disappointing'.

Wilson's recommendations include the provision of an education programme to ensue that the assessment performed by the specialist palliative care nurses is structured. The role of the patient as service user and educator was not included in the proposed education of nurses. The concept of professional and patient partnership has evolved beyond the bounds of clinical practice. It is now widely acknowledged that user involvement in education is both desirable and practicable (Masters *et al.*, 2002).

Carpenter's recommendations focus on an induction programme, leadership, role clarity, and protected team time for team building. While these recommendations are appropriate and reflect the needs of the critical care nurses, they do not go far enough to include measures to promote inter-professional partnership between doctors and nurses, as well as the intensive care unit, outreach and ward nurses.

The success of critical care outreach depends partly on the ability of outreach nurses to work with the ward team, doctors and nurses, as an integrated whole, sharing responsibility and expertise and focusing on the needs of critically ill patients. Inter-professional learning is becoming increasingly recognised as the means to promote teamwork among health care professionals, and forging closer links between health care delivery and health professional education (Wilcock and Headrick, 2000).

Keating makes five recommendations, none of which acknowledge the role of users and informal carers in service planning. In particular, the recommendation for the development of an education programme for nurses depicts a lost opportunity to introduce inter-professional learning to facilitate partnership working among professionals. Critics of team working warn that it is not only important that professionals work together in increasingly flexible and innovative ways, but also that they are required to play formal roles in NHS management and policy (Boaden and Leaviss, 2000). This requirement more than addresses the interpersonal dynamics; it demands a shared understanding of the policy context.

Fear and uncertainty

Fear and uncertainty are emotions shared by participants in Carpenter's and Wilson's studies. The specialist palliative care nurses speak of the first assessment in the community as a daunting experience: '... you don't know what you are going to find out, maybe someone in a lot of pain, maybe someone very angry, very distressed, so a lot of uncertainty'. They are uncertain about what problems/needs the patients might have and how they themselves might react to the patients. They are also aware that just as they are assessing the patients, they themselves are being assessed. The emotional response to this awareness suggests that they see themselves as fallible and patients as capable of forming their own impression. This perspective reflects the attributes of partnership described by Fealy (1995), in that professionals see themselves as equal to the patient.

In Carpenter's study, one of the critical care nurses speaks of being 'scared out of my wits' when fulfilling her new role as a member of the outreach team within an unfamiliar ward setting. She was conscious that she did not 'have the safety net' of the previous intensive care environment. By contrast, one nurse who had recent ward experience felt that she knew 'this place like the back of [her] hand' and experienced less stress. These findings suggest that trust cannot be assumed because of the ideal that nurses should work across organisational boundaries in a holistic way to meet patients' needs. Trust in this instance refers to the expectations held by the critical care nurses that their colleagues in the immediate patient care environment will behave in a particular way that is both predictable and reliable. The tension felt by critical care nurses is testimony to the claim that conventional analysis of partnership working takes for granted the fact that partnership is a 'good thing', and fails to recognise the aforementioned interpersonal dynamics (Grimshaw *et al.*, 2002).

Nonetheless, fear of uncertainty as illustrated in these two studies is not a negative drive. It led to nurses conducting a 'pre-assessment' by studying the referral form before meeting the patient in Wilson's study. This approach prepared the nurses for their first meeting with the patient and enabled them to be sensitive to the main reasons for referral. In Carpenter's study, nurses who felt that they were working outside their safety net worked hard to achieve, and took pride in, a sense of belonging. For example, '... we got invited to a Christmas meal on a ward' was seen as a 'definite' confirmation of acceptance. The effort made by the specialist palliative care nurses to get to know the patients and the effort made by the critical nurses in order to belong to the ward team suggest that both groups of nurses were connecting with their partners, the first of five stages in the life cycle of partnership (http://www.ourpartnership.org.uk/).

For the patient, fear of uncertainty as an unmet emotional need was not helpful. The client focus group in Keating's work revealed that they faced the uncertainty resulting from their stroke totally unprepared. They wanted to understand what had happened to them and how they would continue to be affected on a daily basis. Instead, 'when I go home, like the emotional side, I wasn't told', and 'they want everyone out of hospital and getting better at home and then nobody helps'. These findings confirm that the needs of people who had suffered a stroke are poorly understood and that health and social services continue to ignore stroke survivors' emotional needs. It would seem that patient-centred care remains out of reach for these people and their views are not sought or understood. The implementation of the Department of Health's *National Service Framework for Long-Term Conditions* promotes the role of this group of patients in the management of their own condition and is expected to enhance their partnership status (Department of Health, 2005).

Conflict

The palliative care nurses experienced conflict in their relationship with patients and their families. They often felt pressurised to collude with the family to shield the patient from the diagnosis of cancer and worsening prognosis; yet they also felt duty bound to protect the patient's right to know. They also acknowledged that balancing the conflicting needs of the patient and his or her family was crucial to the maintenance of the therapeutic relationship. The palliative care nurses demonstrated that they were able to work through the conflict by being open, honest and non-judgemental in their communication with the family and patients.

A minority of the critical care nurses experienced conflict in their role as a result of personality clashes, differing team ideology and a lack of consistency in terms of role expectations. The remainder, the majority, did not experience these problems because of openness in their relationship and effective processes being in place for communication and solving team problems.

The service providers in Keating's study talked about the economic pressure that led to their denial of the real needs of the patients. Knowing that their own action and inaction adversely affected the lives of so many people made them feel guilty. Their coping strategy was to focus on specific aspects of the patient separately rather than the person as a whole. They also said 'if they start walking then [I] can move away', which suggests the premature withdrawal of services. The client group in the same study spoke of inconsistency in the service's objective: 'they want everyone to get out of hospital and get better at home, and then nobody helps'. They felt unprepared to cope with life at home and the emotional aftermath of a stroke. These findings demonstrate a service that is not focused on the needs of its client group, and a patient–professional relationship that is not oriented towards partnership working.

Keating's findings also show that there is conflict between the perception of the service providers and the client group. The providers advocated the stroke support group to provide social support and information. The client group did not raise this as an area of need for future service development.

Conflict is inevitable in partnership working (http://www.ourpartnership. org.uk/). The important aspect of partnership is that conflict is managed and resolved. In the palliative care study, the nurses were able to demonstrate this process. There was no evidence of this in the critical care and stroke studies.

Resources

Further analysis of the three papers identifies resource as a consistent theme. The palliative care nurses described the importance of a patient–nurse relationship that is based on intimacy, trust and empathy. This relationship is adversely affected if the nurse who is to carry on working with the patient does not perform the first assessment. Wilson therefore called for sufficient resources (staff and money) to ensure that palliative care nurses can perform the first assessment of patients for whom they have responsibility for ongoing care.

The critical care nurses found that they were not adequately prepared for their new role. While they found the induction programme of two to four weeks essential in reducing the stress level in the early days, the content was not helpful; they therefore did not feel competent to fulfil their role. This feeling, coupled with the initial suspicion and hostility from the ward staff, raised their stress levels. Where leadership was weak and there was poor team cohesion among the critical care nurse outreach team, morale was low. Carpenter recommended that protected time should be provided for team building, professional development and networking in order to build relationships.

Keating found that inadequate resources resulted in unmet needs, particularly the psychosocial needs of individuals recovering from stroke. The research recommended that all patients should be offered an individualised educational programme to enable understanding of stroke. Education and training were also recommended for nurses so that they can work with the patient to enhance self-care capacity. These recommendations have resource implications. The interpersonal conflict identified earlier also requires personal resources (emotion, interpersonal skills and time) if team working is to succeed.

Outcome measures of successful partnership often focus on improvement in effectiveness and efficiency through reductions in duplication and overlap in effort (Burch and Borland, 2001). Such expectation is at odds with the findings of all three studies reviewed; the recommendations of all three studies, if accepted and implemented, will increase the cost of service delivery.

Conclusion

This review of the three papers found that partnership working is costly and fraught with difficulty. When partners first come together and before they get to know one another, they are fearful of uncertainty. The fear experienced by the palliative care nurses is grounded in a very different context from that experienced by the critical care nurses and the client group of the stroke study. This finding supports the view that the context of partnership function is an important determinant of the types and levels of partnership working (Wildridge, 2004). The solution to partnership problems thus needs to be context specific.

All three studies identified conflict in terms of needs and views; this in turn creates interpersonal conflict. Conflict between partners is acknowledged as inevitable; partnership survival depends on its ability to manage and resolve conflict (http://www.ourpartnership.org.uk/). Some of the participants of these three studies have demonstrated skills and commitment to resolve such issues through openness, honesty and non-judgemental communication.

Partnership working is not a soft option to reduce cost; it requires ongoing investment of time, personal effort (interpersonal skills and emotion) and money. Partnership working is taken for granted as a 'good thing', but research evaluation often neglects the wider costs (Grimshaw *et al.*, 2000).

References

Audit Commission (1999) *The Provision of Critical Care Services in England and Wales*. Audit Commission, London.

Ball, C. (ed.) (2002) Critical care outreach services – do they make a difference? *Intensive and Critical Care Nursing*, **18**, 257–60.

Barker, P. (1997) *Assessment in Psychiatric and Mental Health Nursing: In Search of the Whole Person*. Nelson Thornes, London.

Bernard, H. (2000) *Social Research Methods*. Sage Publications, London.

Burgess, R. (1984) *In the Field: An Introduction to Field Research*. Allen & Unwin, London.

Boaden, N. and Leaviss, J. (2000) Putting team work in context. *Medical Education*, **34**, 921–7.

Burch, S. and Borland, C. (2001) Collaboration, facilities and communities in day care services. *Health and Social Care in the Community*, **11**, 85–94.

Burton, C. (2000) Living with stroke: a phenomenological study. *Journal of Advanced Nursing*, **32**(2), 301–9.

Cancer Relief Macmillan Fund (1995) *The Operational Management of a New Home-Based Macmillan Service*. Cancer Relief Macmillan Fund, London.

Cancer Research Campaign (1993) *Assessing Patients with Cancer – The Contents, Skills and Process of Assessment*. Psychological Medicine Group, Manchester.

Carod-Artal, J., Egido, J., Gonzàlez, J. and de Seijas V (2000) Quality of life among stroke survivors evaluated 1 year after stroke. *Stroke*, December, 2996–3000.

Cartledge, S. (2001) Factors influencing the turnover of intensive care nurses. *Intensive and Critical Care Nursing*, **17**, 348–55.

Cavanagh, S. J. (1992) Predictors of nursing staff turnover. *Journal of Advanced Nursing*, **15**, 373–80.

Chellel, A., Fraser, J., Fender, V., Higgs, D., Buas-Rees, S., Hook, L., Cook, C., Parson, S. and Thomas, C. (2002) Nursing observations on ward patients at risk of critical illness. *Nursing Times*, **12**(98), 46.

Collins, K., Jones, M. L., McDonnell, A., Read, S., Jones, R. and Cameron, A. (2000) Do new roles contribute to job satisfaction and retention of staff in nursing and professions allied to medicine? *Journal of Nursing Management*, **8**, 3–12.

Coombs, M. and Dillon, A. (2002) Crossing boundaries, re-defining care: the role of the Critical Care Outreach Team. *Journal of Clinical Nursing*, **11**, 387–93.

Cormack, D. (1996) *The Research Process in Nursing*, 3rd edn. Blackwell Science, Oxford.

Cutcliffe, J., Black, C., Hanson, E. and Goward, P. (2001) The commonality and synchronicity of mental health nurses and palliative care nurses: closer than you think? Parts 1 and 2. *Journal of Psychiatric and Mental Health Nursing*, **8**, 53–66.

Department of Health (1991) *Junior Doctors: The New Deal*. Health Service Management Executive, Department of Health, London.

Department of Health (1997) *The New NHS: Modern and Dependable*. Department of Health, London.

Department of Health (1998) *Modernising Social Services*. Department of Health, London.

Department of Health (1999) *Saving Lives: Our Healthier Nation*. Department of Health, London.

Department of Health (2000a) *Comprehensive Critical Care: A Review of Adult Critical Care Services*. Department of Health, London.

Department of Health (2000b) *The NHS Plan: A Plan for Investment, a Plan for Reform*. Department of Health, London.

Department of Health (2000c) *The NHS Cancer Plan: A Plan for Investment, a Plan for Reform*. Department of Health, London.

Department of Health (2001a) *The Nursing Contribution to the Provision of Comprehensive Care for Adults – A Strategic Programme of Action*. Department of Health, London.

Department of Health (2001b) *National Service Framework for Older People*. Department of Health, London.

Department of Health (2005) *The National Service Framework (NSF) for Long-Term Conditions*. Department of Health, London.

Edwards, A. and Talbot, R. (1997) *The Hard Pressed Researcher*. Longman, London.

Edwards, M. and Miller, C. (2001) Improving psychosocial assessment in oncology. *Professional Nurse*, **16**(7), 223–6.

Fealy, G. M. (1995) Professional caring: the moral dimension. *Journal of Advanced Nursing*, **22**(6), 1135–40.

Franklin, C. and Mathew, J. (1994) Developing strategies to prevent in-hospital cardiac arrest analysing responses of physicians and nurses in the hours before the event. *Critical Care Medicine*, **22**, 244–7.

Freeth, D. (2001) Sustaining inter-professional collaboration. *Journal of Inter-Professional Care*, **15**(1), 37–46.

Geddes, J. and Chamberlain, M. (1994) Improving social outcome after stroke: an evaluation of the volunteer stroke scheme. *Clinical Rehabilitation*, **8**, 116–26.

Glaser, B. and Strauss, A. (1967) *The Discovery of Grounded Theory – Strategies for Qualitative Research*. Aldine, New York.

Glass, T. A. and Maddox, G. L. (1992) The quality and quantity of social support: stroke recovery as psycho-social transition. *Social Science and Medicine*, **34**, 1249–61.

Goldhill, D., White, A. and Sumner, A. (1999) Physiological values and procedures in the 24 hours before ICU admission from the ward. *Anaesthesia*, **54**, 529–34.

Goffman, E. (1970) *Strategic Interaction*. University of Pennsylvania Press, Pennsylvania.

Grimshaw, D., Vincent, S. and Willmott, H. (2002) Going privately: partnership and outsourcing in UK public services. *Public Administration*, **80**(3), 475–502.

Gubrium, J. and Holstein, J. A. (eds.) (2002) *Handbook of Interview Research – Context and Method*. Sage, London.

Hastings, R. (1996) *Developing Questionnaires for Research and Evaluation – a Practical Guide*. Institute for Child Health, London.

Heaven, C. and Maguire, P. (1998) The relationship between patients' concerns and psychological distress in a hospice setting. *Psycho-oncology*, **7**, 502–7.

Henneman, E., Lee, J. and Cohen, J. (1995) Collaboration: a concept of analysis. *Journal of Advanced Nursing*, **21**, 103–9.

Hilton, R. (1995) Fragmentation within inter-professional work: a result of isolationism in health care professional education and the preparation of students to function only in the confines of their own discipline. *Journal of Inter-Professional Care*, **9**(1), 33–40.

James, V. and Field, D. (1996) Who has the power? Some problems and issues affecting the nursing care of dying patients. *European Journal of Cancer Care*, **5**, 73–80.

Joint Consultants' Committee (2002–2003) *Staffing Acute Hospitals at Nights and Weekends: The Role of Competency-based Multidisciplinary Teams.* Joint Consultants' Committee, London.

Jones, A. (1999) A heavy and blessed experience: a psychoanalytic study of community Macmillan nurses and their roles in serious illness and palliative care. *Journal of Advanced Nursing*, **30**(6), 1297–303.

Judd, C., Smith, E. and Kidder, l. (1991) *Research Methods and Social Relations*, 6th edn. Harcourt Brace Jovanovich, London.

Kratz, C. R. (1979) *The Nursing Process.* Baillière Tindall, London.

Keane, A., Duceite, J. and Adler, D. (1985) Stress in intensive care and non-intensive care nurses. *Nursing Research*, **34**(94), 231–6.

Kim, P., Warren, S., Madill, H. and Hadley, M. (1999) Quality of life of stroke survivors. *Quality of Life Research*, **8**, 293–301.

King, R. (1996) Quality of life after stroke. *Stroke*, **27**(9), 1467–72.

Korbasa, S. (1982) Hardiness and health: a prospective study. *Personality and Social Psychology*, **42**(1), 168–77.

Lally, I. and Pearce, J. (1996) Intensive care nurses' perceptions of stress. *Nursing in Critical Care*, **1**(1), 17–25.

Laungani, P. (2002) The counselling interview: first impressions. *Counselling Psychology Quarterly*, **15**(1), 107–13.

Loher, B., Noe, R. A., Moeller, N. L. and Fitzgerald, M. P. (1985) A meta-analysis of the relation of job characteristics to job satisfaction. *Journal of Applied Psychology*, **70**, 280–9.

Masters, H., Forrest, S., Harley, A., Hunter, M., Brown, N. and Risk, I. (2002) Involving mental health service users and carers in curriculum development: moving beyond classroom involvement. *Journal of Psychiatric and Mental Health Nursing*, **9**, 309–16.

Martin, J., Meltzer, H. and Elliot, D. (1988) *The Prevalence of Disability Among Adults.* HMSO, London.

Matthias, P., Prime, R. and Thompson, T. (1997) *Preparation for Inter-Professional Work: Holism, Integration and the Purpose of Training and Education.* Macmillan, Basingstoke.

McQuillan, P., Pilkington, S., Allen, A., Taylor, B., Short, A., Morgan, G., Nielson, M., Barrett, D., Smith, G. and Collin, C. (1998) Confidential inquiry into quality of care before admission to intensive care. *British Medical Journal*, **316**, 1853–8.

Megel, M. and Elrod, M. (1993) Ethical and interpersonal conflicts experienced by nursing QA/QI professionals: justice or care? *Journal of Nursing Care Quality*, **7**(4), 6–18.

National Institute for Clinical Excellence (2004) *Guidance on Cancer Services – Improving Supportive and Palliative Care for Adults with Cancer.* National Institute for Clinical Excellence, London.

North Essex Health Authority (2000) *North Essex Needs Assessment.* North Essex Health Authority (Unpublished)

Oehring, A. and Oakley, J. (1994) The young stroke patient: a need for specialised group support systems. *Topics in Stroke Rehabilitation*, **1**(1), 25–40.

Office for National Statistics (1997) *Mortality Statistics, 1996.* Office for National Statistics, London.

Omery, A. (1983) Phenomenology: a method for nursing research. *Advances in Nursing Science*, **5**(2), 49–63.

Ovretveit, J. (1993) *Co-ordinating Community Care: Multidisciplinary Teams and Care Management.* Open University Press, Buckingham.

Page, S. (1999) *The Shadow and the Counsellor – Working with Darker Aspects of the Person, Role and Profession.* Routledge, Taylor & Francis Group, Oxford.

Polit, D. and Hungler, B. (1997) *Essentials of Nursing Research: Methods, Appraisal, and Utilization*, 4th edn. Lippincott, Philadelphia.

Pollock, S. (1997) A district stroke service. *British Journal of Hospital Medicine*, **57**(5), 224–8.

Pound, P. and Gompertz, P. (1998) A patient centred study of the consequences of stroke. *Clinical Rehabilitation*, **12**, 338–47.

Rawaf, S. and Orton, P. (2000) *Health Improvement Programmes.* Royal Society of Medicine Press, London.

Reed, J. and Roskell-Payton, V. (1997) Focus groups: issues of analysis and interpretation. *Journal of Advanced Nursing*, **26**, 765–71.

Roberts, P. (1997) Planning and running a focus group. *Nurse Researcher*, **4**(4), 78–82.

Ross, C. and Reskin, B. (1992) Education, control at work and job satisfaction. *Social Science Research*, **21**(2), 34–48.

Round, A. (2001) Introduction to clinical reasoning. *Journal of Evaluation in Clinical Practice*, **7**(2), 109–117.

Royal College of Nursing (2003) *Defining Nursing.* http://www.rcn.org. uk/downloads/definingnursing/definingnursing-a4.pdf (Last accessed 14 March 2006).

Sawatzky, J. (1996) Stress in critical care nurses: actual and perceived. *Heart and Lung*, **25**(5), 409–17.

Skilbeck, J. and Seymour, J. (2002) Meeting complex needs: an analysis of Macmillan nurses' work with patients. *International Journal of Palliative Nursing*, **8**(12), 574–82.

Stenhouse, C. (2001) *Outreach: A Guideline for the Introduction of Outreach Services (Draft)*. Intensive Care Society, London.

Stevens, A. and Bickler, G. (2000) Health needs assessment and health improvement programmes. In: *Health Improvement Programmes* (eds. S. Rawaf and P. Orton). Royal Society of Medicine Press, London.

Stevens, A. and Raftery, J. (eds.) (1994) *Health Care Needs Assessment: The Epidemiological Based Needs Assessment Reviews*. Radcliffe Medical Press, Oxford.

Stroke Association, The (1997) *Stroke, National Tragedy, National Priority – An Agenda for Action in Stroke Prevention, Treatment and Care*. The Stroke Association, London.

Stroke Association, The (1998) Stroke care: reducing the burden of disease. The Stroke Association, London.

Swartzman, L., Gibson, M. and Armstrong, T. (1998) Psychosocial considerations in adjustment to stroke. *Physical Medicine and Rehabilitation*, **12**(3), 519–41.

Toghill, P. J. (1994) *Examining Patients – An Introduction to Clinical Medicine*. Edward Arnold, London.

Tomlinson, F. (2005) Idealistic and pragmatic version of the discourse of partnership. *Organisation Studies*, **26**(8), 1169–88.

Trnobranski, P. (1995) Implementation of community care policy in the United Kingdom: will it be achieved? *Journal of Advanced Nursing*, **21**, 998–5.

van den Bos, G. and Triemstra, A. (1999) Quality of life as an instrument for need assessment and outcome assessment of health care in chronic patients. *Quality in Health Care*, **8**, 247–52.

Van Veenendaal, H., Grinspun, D. and Adriaanse, H. (1996) Education needs of stroke survivors and their family members as perceived by themselves and health professionals. *Patient Education and Counselling*, **28**, 265–76.

Weltermann, B., Homann, J., Rogalewski, A., Brach, S., Voss, S. and Ringelstein, E. (2000) Stroke knowledge among stroke groups members. *Stroke*, **31**, 1230–3.

Wilcock, P. M. and Headrick, L. A. (2000) Inter-professional learning for the improvement of health care: why bother? *Journal of Inter-Professional Care*, **14**(2), 111–17.

Wildridge, V., Childs, S., Cawthra, L. and Madge, B. (2004) How to create successful partnerships – a review of the literature. *Health Information and Libraries Journal*, **21**, 3–19.

Wilkinson, J. and Murray, S. (1998) Assessment in primary care: practical issues and possible approaches. *British Medical Journal*, **316**, 1524–8.

Williams, L., Weinberger, M., Harris, L. and Biller, J. (1999) Measuring quality of life in a way that is meaningful to stroke patients. *Neurology*, **53**, 1839–43.

World Health Organization (1987) *People's Needs for Nursing Care: A European Study: A Study of Nursing Care Needs and of the Planning, Implementation and Evaluation of Care Provided by Nurses in Two Selected Groups of People in the European Region.* WHO Regional Office for Europe, Geneva.

Wright, D. (2001) Hospice nursing – the speciality. *Cancer Nursing*, **24**(1), 20–7.

CHAPTER 6

Implications for future partnerships

Part 1
Implications for future partnerships in psychiatric care
Peter J. Martin

Intentions

* To examine common partnership themes within a psychiatric context
* To make recommendations for developing partnerships in psychiatric care

Introduction

The papers contained in this book provide insight into the scope of partnerships in health care. They suggest that the term *partnership* is not condensed into a single pithy statement; instead, it is a dynamic concept demonstrated through the practice of nurses who have provided papers for this book. This may be preferable: instead of applying a single 'one size fits all approach' the writers have demonstrated that each work differently, but there are discernable themes that can be ascribed as 'partnership'.

This paper revisits and expands upon some of the ground covered within the introductory chapter. Partnership with service users and partnership between service providers was presented as a positive aspiration, but problematic to achieve in practice. From the reviews of the nine papers within this book, common partnership themes have emerged. These themes have been grouped under the broad headings of context of partnership, health care workers and partnership outcomes, which form the basis of this discussion.

Context of partnership

The context in which partnerships were developed was noted to be significant. It was demonstrated through the papers in terms of organisational culture, the authority of professions within health care, the perception of a supportive environment and change (Onyett, 2005, p. 97):

> Clearly, effective working relationships between staff and service users do not in themselves create good mental health services. They provide the necessary, if not sufficient, condition for an environment in which users, their social networks and staff can work together to achieve the best outcome given the prevailing conditions.

Organisational culture

Many of the papers presented in this book discussed 'context' as the prevailing organisational culture that must be healthy for partnerships to flourish, a view supported by Hickey and Kipping (1998). An organisation may espouse the benefits of partnership and give overt encouragement to staff to work in partnership with others. However, the covert message may be one that encourages people to be passive and non-innovating, enabling the status quo to be maintained throughout the organisation. People may be discouraged from innovating if punishment and blame are perceived as the consequence of change. Eastbrook's and Reynolds' papers emphasise the importance of an organisation presenting a congruent message both overtly and covertly to staff and service users about the importance of partnership.

Before service users and health care workers can work in partnership the organisation must support multi-professional and multi-agency partnerships. Health care workers cannot engage service users in partnership if they do not feel empowered or if they feel compromised by poor relationships with other members of the team (Hickey and Kipping, 1998). The context that Wrycraft described as existing within the Trail Blazers course supported partnership working between service providers. This culture was multi-professional but relatively power-neutral, with participants sharing a common outcome.

Professions

Treadwell and Young note that professions remain a dominant force within the patient's experience of health care. This dominance is a significant aspect of the entire health system and shapes the organisational culture within which health care is delivered. Professional dominance may be seen as a positive or negative force, depending on how the relationship between professional and society is understood (Gabe *et al.*, 2004). In many of the papers professional dominance was a hurdle to partnership between service providers and between service providers and service users.

Ensuring the right interpersonal relations remains important, as Carpenter noted; good interpersonal relationships and respect within teams promote healthy partnerships. The development of multi-professional working within the health care team is essential if partnerships are to be realised. Partnerships require relationships within multi-professional teams to be collaborative and based upon equality and respect rather than riven by inter-professional rivalry and personality conflicts. However, there remains an attachment to uni-professional cultures, supported by differences in education, status and financial reward (Norman and Peck, 1999). Such an attachment acts as a barrier to effective multi-professional working. Professional education should examine real-world problems of team working and recognise that diversity might be preferable to a universal prescriptive model (Stark *et al.*, 2002). Treadwell and Keating's papers both discuss professionalism within the health system.

Within teams Keating noted that professionals focused on part of the patient rather than the whole. This allowed professionals to withdraw services early where resources were limited. Looking at the person as a collection of systems may be a defence against the anxiety of being with people in distress or reveal the continued dominance of the primarily reductionist medical model. In Treadwell's paper, professionalism alienates patients from involvement and engagement with the services. Treadwell also noted that, for partnerships with service users to be effective, professionals needed to be sensitive to the patient and adopt a respectful non-judgemental attitude that acknowledged them as individuals.

There are many aspects of professionalism that are desirable within the health services. These may include the underpinning desire to do what is right and to be personally accountable for what is done. Similarly, professionalism can lead to disrespect, lack of concern for the individual and the alienation of the individual. The papers in this book have highlighted the importance of achieving a service which is of the highest professional quality but which is also service user focused.

Support

In the psychiatric services the move to a community-based setting has changed the support networks that existed within institutions. Carpenter noted that health care workers in supportive team environments are more able to work in partnerships with service users.

Treadwell identified that a lack of trust existed between service users and service providers which had a damaging effect on the development of partnerships. Trust within partnerships, between service users and the health care workers, parallels the support and trust experienced within the multi-professional team. In contemporary psychiatric practice health care workers are expected to provide a relationship that empowers people, promoting safety alongside positive risk taking (Department of Health, 2004). They may feel exposed and in a 'risky' position leading to stress and anxiety that must be resolved (Rose *et al.*, 2004). If this is not resolved through the use of support networks the ability to manage further risks in service user partnerships may be hampered and ineffective. The significance of supervision as a component of a supportive service to ameliorate stress and anxiety was a factor to which Wilson drew attention.

The papers in this book highlight that the environment in which partnerships occur must be supportive, with attention paid to the well-being, growth and development of team members (Sainsbury Centre for Mental Health, 2000).

Change

The change process appears directly or indirectly in all the papers. Partnership working requires fundamental change in the relationship between all the participants in health care. In contemporary psychiatric care services, users want a better partnership of care with professionals (Sainsbury Centre for Mental Health, 1994); such demands, previously perceived as revolutionary, are now largely accepted practice. The organisation of service users within user groups and the activities of these groups, as well as individuals, have contributed significantly to the rapid redistribution of power within the system. Nonetheless, this change begins from a state of powerlessness, so people with mental illness continue to be disempowered and to experience poverty and discrimination within communities (see Campbell, 2005). Wildridge *et al.* (2004) note that if a partnership starts out on the basis of unequal power then the most powerful partner will get the greatest benefit and the least powerful will incur a larger burden of costs.

In conclusion, the sort of context in which partnerships will flourish is one that is transparent and supportive. The creation of partnerships and effective partnership working are hampered by unhealthy cultures in which professional hegemonies and poor management of stress abound. It requires a stronger emphasis on shared values and practice that crosses professional divides and a stronger recognition of the importance of the local organisational culture (Onyett, 2005).

Health care workers

Working in partnership – developing and maintaining constructive working relationships with service users, carers, families, colleagues, lay people and wider community networks. Working positively with any tensions created by conflicts of interest or aspiration that may arise between the partners in care. (Department of Health, 2004, p. 3)

Communication

The health care worker seeks partnership with other service providers and with service users. Both expressions of partnership require effective communication.

The health care worker communicates knowledge to the service users; this knowledge might include, for example, details about medical tests, as in Eastbrook's and Reynolds' studies. To other service providers it might be a unique professional perspective on the service user's care. In order to communicate knowledge the health care worker must be committed to seeking out information and communicating effectively. Eastbrook's and Reynolds' studies have shown that nurses did not access information in a timely and efficient manner, nor did they communicate the information to service users. Furthermore, Carpenter's study identifies how professional boundaries can adversely impact upon effective communication. As was identified by Eastbrook and Reynolds, nurses avoided communicating with patients, thus creating unnecessary fear and uncertainty for service users and carers. Narrowing the information gap between partners is essential if partnerships are to exist (Cahill, 1996).

Dissemination of knowledge is an activity integral to partnerships; it is also bi-directional. Health care workers need to provide adequate space and time to enable service users and carers to inform, to question and to clarify information. In order to facilitate this exchange health care workers must respect and value the information that is provided by users and carers. This will enable service users to play an active role in the development of their own care plan and decisions about their health needs. Listening to what service users and carers have to say is not always comfortable, nor may details of preferred lifestyle or aspirations seem immediately relevant, but it is important in establishing and maintaining partnerships (Department of Health, 2004). The subjective experience of service users is valued for authenticity, but when set beside evidence-based knowledge the authenticity occupies second place (Rose *et al.*, 2004). The participants in Young's study reported that there was a lack of support from health care workers because of a lack of understanding of the individual's quality of life. If professionals do not believe service users' views to be valid or important then the involvement of service users in decision making is severely restricted (Hickey and Kipping, 1998).

If health care workers do not communicate knowledge and understanding of the service user to multi-professional and multi-agency teams, the service user cannot benefit from effective team working. The team must provide the space to listen to each other and to respect what is disseminated. Members of multi-professional or multi-agency teams may come from diverse backgrounds and bring potentially conflicting information. Partnership working requires individuals and teams to work positively and determine how to overcome such difficulties and to reap the benefits of working in partnership (Department of Health, 2004).

In order to engage in effective communication the health care worker should possess the appropriate communication skills. Interpersonal skills and a positive attitude, although not unique to nurses, are perceived as crucial to their work (Peck and Norman, 1999). Some of the papers in this book suggest that nurses did not consider communication to be important in relation to the more technical aspects of their work. Skilled communication should be fundamental to psychiatric care, and similar skills should be applied to improving partnership working with service users and in other partnerships. Despite this, problems with both the content and the process of communication continue to be reported (National Institute for Mental Health in England, 2003).

The health care worker requires an attitude toward communication that emphasises the importance of the task and the significant contribution that it makes to the user's experience. Eastbrook's and Reynolds' studies both showed that the nurses in the samples had a distorted perception of communication. If partnerships are to operate effectively, health care workers should regard the service user as an information hub rather than the end of a long chain of information exchanges.

A multi-professional team cannot function if members regard information as personal and professional property. The team should regard information as equally valuable and available to each member of the team. There is no room for professions to become precious about specific information or to feel professionally compromised if information is incomplete as in Eastbrook's and Reynolds' studies. Professionals continue to develop in professional silos where professional prestige is paramount. To work effectively in partnerships professional barriers must be destroyed and replaced by good quality communication.

Confidence

Health care workers need to have confidence in their professional role in order to contribute to partnership working. This confidence is related to the environment in which they function. A healthy organisational culture, supportive of partnership working, will enhance professional confidence and the quality of care. Professional confidence is sapped where 'powerful' professionals disregard the contributions of others and work occurs in isolation.

The confidence of health care workers to engage in partnerships may also be affected by the perception that service users will be critical of the care that they have delivered (Higgins, 1994). Reynolds' and Treadwell's papers both referred to nurses being negatively evaluated by patients and carers.

In conclusion, if health care workers are to participate in and support partnership working they need to be able to communicate effectively with other and have the confidence in their worker contribution.

Partnership outcomes

In the health care team the return of service users to their former health state may be an implicit shared outcome, but the manner in which this may be achieved is not always effectively shared. The multiplicity of ideologies that exist within the psychiatric services, for example: psychiatrists, nurses, social workers, voluntary groups, can have the effect of destabilising effective partnership working (Wildridge *et al.*, 2004). It is essential that the team demonstrate shared values as the basis of partnerships, whilst recognising the individual contribution that each member makes. This was demonstrated in Wrycraft's work with the assertive outreach team.

If service users and service providers are to invest time and energy into partnerships, there must be some benefit associated with the activity (Cahill, 1996). The outcome for service providers is in attaining shared goals and Wrycraft's work on the Trail Blazers project demonstrated how this could be achieved. The outcome of partnerships with service users is underpinned also by shared goals, but as Wrycraft's work on assertive outreach describes, goals can be quite different. The papers do not provide an answer to this dilemma, which, as was noted in the introduction, presents a serious challenge to working in partnership within a psychiatric context.

The assumption that has underpinned this discussion is that service users wish to be partners in their care. There are occasions when service users want to hand over decision making to health care workers in whom they trust (Hickey and Kipping, 1998). This remains congruent with the idea of partnership provided it is a temporary measure and based upon informed judgement.

A 'sleeping partner' within the partnership between service users and health care workers is the wider society. The health care worker must work within a framework defined by the current perspective that society has of mental illness. Lack of understanding and fear of mental illness ensure that the boundary defined by society as marking what is acceptable and what is unacceptable behaviour is in continual motion.

Conclusion

Partnership is a policy direction that is unlikely to change in the foreseeable future and, as such, has been the subject of an emergent literature. The papers in this book have demonstrated how partnership is delivered in primary, secondary and tertiary care services. These papers have examined partnerships in real world settings delivered by real world practitioners. Three themes have been found to be common across the different settings: context of partnership, health care workers and partnership outcomes.

Whilst there are many examples of partnership working well, and with the support of health care providers and service users, there is a backdrop of services that espouse, but do not engage with, partnership. Changing attitudes requires cultural shifts throughout the health services. The papers in this book have pointed to some approaches that could be adopted to bring about such change. The approaches support many of the recommendations made, within a psychiatric context, in previous work such as *Taking Your Partners* (Sainsbury Centre for Mental Health, 2000), *Pulling Together* (Sainsbury Centre for Mental Health, 2000) and *Cases for Change* (National Institute for Mental Health in England, 2003).

- **Inter-professional and inter-agency working**: The papers in this book have indicated that there is no single way of approaching partnership working. The imposition of a rigid model is unlikely to be effective. Therefore, organisations need to ensure that the right conditions exist for developing partnership working. These conditions have been shown to include respect, equality, support and change. Such aspirations should not be assumed to underpin all health organisations.
- **Inter-professional and inter-agency education**: Wrycraft's evaluation of the Trail Blazer project demonstrates the efficacy of inter-professional and inter-agency working. The model developed ensures that partners have a vested interest in working together to resolve real-world problems. Educating people for the practical problems of team working, rather than just dealing with broad principles, will improve inter-professional and inter-agency working.
- **User involvement in service planning and development**: Service user involvement at the level of planning and development will ensure that services are constructed for people rather than for professionals.

- **User involvement in education**: Eastbrook, Reynolds, Young and Wilson's papers suggest that service users are excluded from partnership working. Changing the attitudes of professionals should be addressed at all educational levels with the sustained and resolute involvement of service users in education.

Part 2
Implications of study findings for future partnerships in health care
Kimmy Eldridge

Intention

- To examine common partnership themes within a UK health care setting
- To make recommendations for developing partnerships in health care

Introduction

This chapter discusses the implications of the themes identified earlier in all nine papers. With the exception of Wrycraft's, all papers were based on small-scale research projects completed as part of an MSc programme. None of the studies had set out to examine partnership working. However, for the purpose of this book, partnership principles were applied to identify common themes. The findings reveal the extent to which partnership working exists within contemporary practice. The common themes are grouped as follows:

- Values
  - Research design
  - Shared aims
  - Trust
- Resources
  - Personal
  - Professional
  - Physical

These themes are not separate entities, but are interconnected. The following discussion will focus on the implications for patients, health care professionals and organisations in future partnership development within the general health care setting.

Values

Research design

The researchers of all seven studies have adopted a qualitative design to address their research questions. In choosing to do so, they have given their patients a voice. The participants of Young's study describe the constraints of living with diabetes and the effect of insulin on their quality of life; the patients of Treadwell's study recounted their struggle to stop smoking and their interaction with health care professionals in this regard. Young and Treadwell have intentionally avoided making any assumptions about the determining features of quality of life associated with diabetes or the psychological factors that predict relapses to smoking. Instead they have sought to describe and understand the issues from the perspective of their patients. This approach acknowledges the importance of the individual's experience, which in turn leads to the collection and analysis of the experiences in the form of narrative with the view to informing practice.

This emphasis on valuing and recognising the contribution of patients and carers is also evident in Eastbrook's and Reynold's studies. Their findings enable improvement of patient care. All four researchers are demonstrating one of the key elements of partnership: improved and enhanced access to services for users and carers (McLaughlin, 2004; Wildridge *et al.*, 2004) and one of the critical success factors of partnership working: acknowledgement of the need for partnership (Hardy *et al.*, 2000).

Similarly, qualitative research design enables Carpenter, Keating and Wilson, who have a managerial role in the health service, to go beyond consulting staff in service planning. They have contextualised the real world in which service users and providers deliver and experience care. The service users and providers of Young's study describe living with the aftermath of stroke and the interaction between patients and professionals in a health service that is under increased resource pressure. Nurses in Carpenter's and Wilson's studies expressed personal and inter-personal conflicts as they performed a new role in a different practice environment and undertook first assessment, respectively.

Qualitative research design as illustrated in these studies embraces the principles of partnership. However, qualitative research is perceived to be inferior to quantitative studies (McPherson and Leydon, 2002; Silverman, 2001). Evidence-based medicine ranks the value of clinical research on a hierarchy; findings from systematic reviews of multiple well-designed randomised controlled trials sit on the top; and in descending order of credibility, qualitative studies has been placed on the bottom (Belsey and Snell, 2001). A randomised control trial, as a quantitative research approach, that focuses on quantifying variables, randomisation and statistical calculation (Cheek *et al.*, 2004) has no place for the subjective experience of patients and negates partnership with the participants (McPherson and Leydon, 2002). In the drive toward evidence-based health care practice, the continuing high regard for randomised control trials at the expense of qualitative studies will prevent the realisation of user involvement in research.

Shared aims

Notwithstanding the lack of clarity in the use of the term 'partnership', analysis of the papers suggests that the lack of shared goals based on common understanding remains a barrier to partnership development. Health professionals often assume that they know their patients and act in their best interests. Such assumptions led doctors in Yung's study to prescribe insulin therapy without concordance. In Treadwell's study this caused the nurse to suggest postponing stopping smoking until after the Christmas and New Year celebrations, a time considered by the nurse to be more suitable.

Eastbrook's study also found that nurses make assumptions about patients' knowledge. No attempt was made to understand what patients really wanted. These findings are evidence that a paternalistic approach to patient care is being practised despite the current emphasis on partnership working. The literature suggests that the lack of shared treatment aims between patient and professional is not isolated or peculiar to local practice (Britten *et al.*, 2000; Henwood *et al.*, 2003).

The lack of understanding and the absence of a shared aim may be the result of patients adopting a passive role, and not telling the professionals what they want from the consultation (Britten *et al.*, 2000). However, patients such as John in Treadwell's study who knew what he wanted, that is, to continue not to smoke, was challenged by the nurse who wanted 'proof' that his intention not to smoke was genuine. Henwood *et al.* (2003) found numerous examples of women who were knowledgeable about their health condition, and who tried but failed to negotiate treatment options with their GPs. They showed that such situations are most common when there is disagreement between 'lay' and medical knowledge, and where a certain level of compliance with medical opinion is required. Extreme cases of this incongruence between what the doctor wants and what patients want have resulted in legal redress; recent examples include a disabled man who was successful in his court battle, as a result of which doctors will have to provide life support when his condition deteriorates (Dyer, 2004). The parents of a young baby failed to overturn a ruling that gave doctors the clinical and legal rights not to resuscitate when the baby's heart stopped (Dyer, 2005).

In an attempt to promote shared decision making, the *British Medical Journal* published a new web site 'Best Treatments' (http://www.besttreatments. co.uk/) in, 2003. This is a significant development because, traditionally, web sites are generally developed separately for doctors and patients. This web site provides both doctors and patients with the same information about the effectiveness of treatments for chronic medical conditions, presented separately within the same site for doctor and patient audiences and drawn from the same evidence sources (Nash *et al.*, 2003). However, accessing this web site will depend on the patients' ability and confidence to surf the internet and make sense of the information. In addition, using this information in their negotiation with health care professionals demands yet another level of confidence and skills. Patients will have to overcome barriers, such as embarrassment or appearing foolish (Wensing and Grol, 1998).

Observers argue that it is not always possible for patients and health care professionals to have the same views about treatment (Marinker and Shaw, 2003; Dudley, 2004). The recent high-profile case in which seven women with early breast cancer successfully demanded Herceptin from the NHS to save their lives illustrates the emotive position of the patients, and the perspective of the doctors when considering treatment such as Herceptin which has yet to be proved effective and has not been licensed for use in early breast cancer (Collier, 2006). It is still accepted that the medical consultant takes responsibility for patient outcomes, both professionally and legally, and therefore it is ultimately his or her decision what treatment is instigated (Dudley, 2004; Gordhandas, 2004). In the case of Herceptin and the seven women in question, the initial decision to decline the drug was over turned after high publicity. Their success illustrates the power and importance of patients' views and the increasing involvement of society at large in health decisions (Collier, 2006).

Supporters of the concept of concordance assert that when disagreement exists, the patient's view should take precedence even though this decision may raise questions about choice and responsibility (Marinker and Shaw, 2003). Shared goals through concordance will require professionals to be open and skilful in explaining the risks and benefits of each treatment option, and patients must accept the uncertainty of health care outcomes, such as the unproven outcomes of Herceptin, including its unknown side effects. Such behaviours on the part of the patient and the professional will be influenced by the policy and politics of the NHS as well as the wider social context. Policy makers and patients will have to accept that longer consultation will be required for this type of patient–professional interaction, and as a result, patients will have to wait longer to be seen and treated. Patients will also have to be ready for such participation and the professionals will need to be willing and able to engage with patients in this way.

Current evidence indicates that doctors have yet to develop the skills of patient-centred consultation, and to consider the patient as a person within his or her individual psychosocial context (Campion *et al.*, 2002). They are still basing their decisions on unchecked assumptions about patients; Britten *et al.* (2000) find that doctors are unaware of patients' views of medication and anxieties about symptoms and treatment. They are unaware that the patient has changed the dosage of their medication (Britten *et al.*, 2000). Added to this there are concerns that nursing is dominated by a technological and prescribed approach to care (Kitson, 2002), and that doctors view patients as problems to be solved. This is moving away from relating to patients in a caring way (Frank, 2002). Charles-Jones *et al.* (2003) argued that as highly qualified nurses in nurse practitioner roles are increasingly working like doctors, focusing on biomedical problems and making diagnoses, they are risking and compromising the holistic nature and high level of personal care inherent in nursing. Intrinsic in the value of partnership is the diversity of knowledge and skills of the partners, as demonstrated in Wrycraft's papers. The differing perspectives of the multi-professional and multi-agency group enable understanding of the issues from a range of standpoints. The observation that nurses are increasingly working like doctors is a potential weakness of a primary care team consisting of doctors and nurses.

The Government is investing £73 million in the training of junior doctors as part of the measures to modernise medical careers (Department of Health, 2005). The new way of delivering postgraduate medical education includes the establishment of a competence-based curriculum for the Foundation Programme of junior doctors. Previously known as pre-registration house officers and senior house officers, junior doctors will now be called Foundation Year one and Year two doctors. The new curriculum is addressing some of the skill gaps. It is explicit in the curriculum that doctors will be able to 'check on patient understanding, concerns and expectation', 'give clear information and encourage questions' and 'take decisions and act with the patient and not for them' (Foundation Programme Committee, 2005). The financial investment and the focus on acting with and not for the patient suggest consistency between education policy and curriculum planning. The outcomes will depend on local implementation.

Keating's study found that the lack of joined-up thinking at organisational level leads to stroke patients being discharged from hospital without adequate care in the community. For the same reason, critical care outreach nurses experience tension with their colleagues in the ward setting, the very group their role is designed to benefit. These findings of Young's and Keating's studies indicate that partnership working at organisational level remains problematic; those with responsibility to make policy and those who are charged to implement it have yet to achieve shared aims. Critics suggest that partnership in the NHS, such as critical care outreach, is centrally driven and, as such, lacks some of the critical success factors (Tailby *et al.*, 2004); e.g. in the case of the critical care outreach study, acknowledgement of the need for partnership and commitment and ownership (Hardy *et al.*, 2000).

Diversity of partners' interests is inevitable. However, the lessons learnt from the studies presented in this book indicate that partnership development as a change process should be carefully managed to reflect partnership principles. This responsibility rests with policy makers, managers, health professionals and the public at large as service users.

Trust

Trust is a strong theme shared by most of the papers. Trust refers to the expectations held by critical care nurses that their colleagues in the immediate patient care environment will behave in a particular way that is both predictable and reliable. For John in Treadwell's study, trust means that he can rely on nurses to support him in his endeavour to give up cigarettes and not to humiliate him in front of his child. In Eastbrook's study, patients trust nurses to provide them with information so that they can give informed consent and plan their day around the investigations. Such trust is based on mutual understanding. Not understanding and knowing their patients' needs results in the nurses of Treadwell's study being unable to meet John's needs. Palliative care nurses describe the importance of getting to know the patient through spending time and communicating effectively.

Eastbrook's study reported patients' anxiety about diagnostic tests about which they had minimal information. Nurses themselves showed little awareness of patients' need for information at the time when they were informed that they needed to have a specific test. This lack of understanding resulted in patients' needs being unmet. Inherent within the concept of patient-centred care is the principle that care is tailored to meet specific needs. Such an approach is based on mutual understanding between the patient and the professional. The findings of Eastbrook and Treadwell also demonstrated nurses' lack of empathy with their patients. Empathy in this context refers to nurses' skill of demonstrating understanding of patients' feelings; in the Treadwell and Eastbrook studies, as nurses' empathy decreased, patients' anxiety increased.

Ultimately, interpersonal trust in a partnership relationship is determined by the commitment of the partners, and their willingness to spend time to get to know each other. Nurses in Carpenter's and Wilson's studies who value their relationship with their colleagues and patients respectively have been able to gain trust.

Resources

Resources emerge as a strong theme in partnership working; and in this context, resources include personal, professional and physical dimensions.

Personal resources

The critical care and palliative care nurses articulated their fear of the unknown and the pressure to perform; for the critical care nurses their fear related to working outside their comfort zone, the intensive care unit and their high expectations of the role, as well as the perceptions of ward staff. The palliative care nurses worry about the unknown nature of patients' needs and expectations. Both these groups of nurses also experienced personal and inter-personal conflicts. The critical care nurses are able to draw on personal resources to confront their differences in a constructive manner. The palliative care nurses take time to prepare for their first meeting with their patients, and through anticipating needs they reduce the uncertainty associated with meeting the patient for the first time. Critical care nurses are able to make ward staff feel less threatened by acknowledging the difficulties that ward staff experience. By contrast, the service providers of Keating's study cope with the resource pressure by premature withdrawal from patients, leaving them with unmet needs. Nurses in Treadwell's study also lacked the personal resource to reflect and be self-aware of the impact of their interaction with patients.

Eastbrook and Reynolds found that barriers to effective information-giving to patients and carers are more than workload and time issues. Nurses appear to be unable to mobilise personal resources to acquire the appropriate knowledge and understanding in order to be able to provide timely and accurate information to patients, a core function of nursing (McCabe, 2004).

Professional resources

Eastbrook and Reynolds identified that nurses were unable to empower patients and carers because they themselves were disempowered. Empowerment refers to the transferring of knowledge and skills to patients to increase their competence, confidence and control (Kennedy *et al.*, 2005). The prerequisites of patient empowerment are professional competence and confidence. Nurses in Eastbrook's and Reynold's studies were not competent in assessing patients' and carers' information needs, and patients reported that nurses were too busy to talk to them. These findings are supported by the literature (Myers, 2001;

McCabe, 2004) and indicate that the problem is more than just poor communication – it is a matter of professional practice. The key attributes of professionals have been identified as (Hilton and Slotnick, 2005):

- Ethical practice
- Reflection and self-awareness
- Commitment to excellence through lifelong learning
- Respect for patients
- Working with others
- Social responsibility

The nurse in Treadwell's study who made John feel humiliated in front of his
daughter demonstrated a lack of respect for John and illustrated unethical practice. Similarly, nurses in Eastbrook's and Reynold's studies lack professional
resource-knowledge and attitudes congruent with ethical practice. The aforementioned finding of the lack of professional resources is a consistent theme shared
by most papers reviewed for the purpose of this book. The service providers of
Keating's needs assessment acknowledge that their narrow focus on part of the
person rather than meeting the needs of the whole person is an issue; nonetheless they continue with such practice. A multi-professional, multi-agency focus
group as part of the needs assessment process enables them to begin talking
about engaging other service organisations and groups in a different way. Sharing their knowledge of these agencies leads to new understanding. In this respect,
knowledge as a professional resource helps to build partnerships.

Nonetheless, the findings of unethical behaviours and the lack of professional resources raise issues about the effectiveness of professional revalida-
tion and investment in continuing professional development. Although these are
legitimate concerns, it is acknowledged that the NHS is a complex organisation
and that changes in professional practice take time to permeate.

Physical resources

The lack of physical resources also impacted upon the implementation of policy
initiatives. Both Carpenter's and Wrycraft's Trail Blazers evaluation identified
the need for resource investment if such developments were to succeed. The
critical care nurses reported that they were not prepared for their new role, and
the researcher recommended the provision of protected time for team building. Participants in Trail Blazers' evaluation also identified protected time as
'thinking space'. Staff time is an expensive resource, but in terms of partnership
development it is an unavoidable expenditure. The findings of Carpenter, Wilson
and Wrycraft indicate that resource issues have not been clearly identified in the

planning of partnership projects. For example, in Carpenter's study, organisations had not developed new structures and processes to support partnership working in outreach work; this lack of a management and support structure had resulted in a lack of role clarity which in turn affected staff morale. In Wilson's study lack of time and resources meant that the initial multi-disciplinary assessment tended to be carried out by nurses alone.

Conclusion

Applying partnership principles to identify common themes from students' existing MSc work has revealed contemporary partnership practice. The implications for future partnership development for patients, professionals and organisations in the general health care setting have been considered from the perspective of values and resources; the theme of values is further divided into three categories: research design, shared aims and trust; while resources contains three dimensions: personal, professional and physical resources.

The findings reveal that nurses as researchers readily embrace partnership principles when employing qualitative study designs. However, the current drive to practice evidence-based health care devalues descriptive evidence. The continuing high regard for randomised control trials hinders the realisation of user involvement in health care research.

The thematic analysis also found a lack of progress in partnership working between patient and professional. The lack of shared aims remains a major barrier. As no two patients respond to the same treatment in an identical way, treatment outcomes remain uncertain. The achievement of concordance will depend on the patients' willingness and ability to engage in the debate about the uncertainty of health care outcomes. Professionals will have to acquire the skills of communicating risk, and explaining treatment options in language that is understandable by the public at large. The Government is making considerable investment in postgraduate medical education to ensure that doctors are able to meet not only the needs of today's patients, but also the needs of tomorrow's health service. However, health services are delivered by multi-professional teams. Unless similar investment is made for the education of nurses and allied health professionals the impact on patient and professional partnership will be compromised.

Other factors that act as barriers to partnership with patients include the lack of personal and professional resources, including the knowledge and skills of nurses. The findings of some of the papers reviewed uncover evidence that nurses lack empathy with patients and self-awareness of their own level of skills and knowledge. Patients found nurses more concerned with performing tasks than communicating with patients. The focus on tasks and the lack of empathy is more than poor communication; it is a lack of professionalism.

The findings further reveal that organisations are implementing government policy without adequate planning and do not have the infrastructure in place to support new partnership working. Nonetheless, projects such as critical care and assertive outreach are successful despite resource constraints because of the personal commitment of the people involved. Future successful patient–professional partnerships and multi-agency and multi-professional collaborations require more than the commitment of a collective few; they are contingent upon a facilitative policy framework, real financial support, time, knowledge, skills and commitment to creating a new structure and managing change.

References

Belsey, J. and Snell, T. (2001) What is evidence-based medicine? *Evidence-Based Medicine*, **1**(2), 1–6; http://www.jr2.ox.ac.uk/bandolier/booth/glossary/EBM.html (accessed 29 March 2006).

Britten, N., Stevenson, F. A., Barry, C., Barber, N. and Bradley, C. P. (2000) Misunderstandings in prescribing decisions in general practice: qualitative study. *British Medical Journal*, **320**(7233), 484–8.

Charles-Jones, H., Latimer, J. and May, C. (2003) Transforming general practice: the redistribution of medical work in primary care. *Sociology of Health and Illness*, **25**(1), 71–92.

Campbell, P. (2005) From little acorns – the mental health service user movement. In: *Beyond the Water Towers* (eds. A. Bell and P. Lindley). London: Sainsbury Centre for Mental Health.

Cahill, J. (1996) Patient participation: a concept analysis. *Journal of Advanced Nursing*, **24**, 561–71.

Campion, P., Foulkes, J., Neighbour, R. and Tate, P. (2002) Patient centredness in the MRCGP video examination: analysis of large cohort. *British Medical Journal*, **325**, 691–2.

Cheek, J., Onslow, M. and Cream, A. (2004) Beyond the divide: comparing and contrasting aspects of qualitative and quantitative research approaches. *Advances in Speech-Language Pathology*, **6**(3), 147–52.

Collier, J. (2006) Panorama: Herceptin – wanting the wonder drug. *British Medical Journal*, **332**, 368.

Department of Health (2004) *The Ten Essential Shared Capabilities*. Department of Health, London.

Department of Health (2005) *£73 Million for Junior Doctor Training Programme*. Press release 2005/0135. Department of Health, London.

Dudley, N. (2004) Dialysis on demand while judges play god. *British Medical Journal*, Rapid reponse to Dyer (2004): `http://bmj.bmjjournals.com/cgi/eletters/329/7461/309#70363` (accessed 5 June 2006).

Dyer, C. (2004) Man wins battle to keep receiving life support. *British Medical Journal*, **329**, 309.

Dyer, C. (2005) Parent fails to overturn ruling not to resuscitate baby. *British Medical Journal*, **330**, 985.

Frank, A. W. (2002) Relations of caring: demoralisation and remoralisation in the clinic. *International Journal for Human Caring*, **6**(2), 13–19.

Foundation Programme Committee (2005) *Curriculum for the Foundation Years in Postgraduate Education and Training*. Foundation Programme Committee of the Academy of Medicinal Royal Colleges in co-operation with Modernising Medical Careers in the Departments of Health. Department of Health, London.

Gabe, J., Bury, M. and Elston, M. (2004) *Key Concepts in Medical Sociology*. Sage, London.

Gordhandas, A. M. (2004) Law is an ass. *British Medical Journal*, Rapid reponse to Dyer(2004):`http://bmj.bmjjournals.com/cgi/eletters/329/7461/309#70664` (accessed 5 June 2006).

Hardy, B., Hudson, B. and Waddington, E. (2000) *What Makes a Good Partnership? A Partnership Assessment Tool*. Leeds: Nuffield Institute for Health.

Henwood, F., Wyatt, S., Hart, A. and Smith, J. (2003) 'Ignorance is bliss sometimes': constraints on the emergence of the 'informed patient' in the changing landscapes of health information. *Sociology of Health and Illness*, **25**(6), 589–607.

Hickey, G. and Kipping, C. (1998) Exploring the concept of user involvement in mental health through a participation continuum. *Journal of Clinical Nursing*, **7**(1), 83–8.

Higgins, R. (1994) Involving users in health care. *Health Services Management*, 14–15 March.

Hilton, S. R. and Slotnick, H. B. (2005) Proto-professionalism: how professionalisation occurs across the continuum of medical education. *Medical Education*, **39**, 58–65.

Kennedy, A., Gask, L. and Rogers, A. (2005) Training professionals to engage with and promote self-management. *Health Education Research*, **20**(5), 567–78.

Kitson, A. (2002) Recognising relationship: reflection on evidence-based practice. *Nursing Inquiry*, **9**(3), 179–86.

McCabe, C. (2004) Nurse–patient communication: an exploration of patients' experience. *Journal of Clinical Nursing,* **13**, 41–9.

Marinker, M. and Shaw, J. (2003) Not to be taken as directed. *British Medical Journal,* **326**, 348–9.

McLaughlin, H. (2004) Partnership: panacea or pretence? *Journal of Inter-Professional Care,* **18**(2), 103–13.

McPherson, K. and Leydon, G. (2002) Quantitative and qualitative methods in UK health research: then, now and....? *European Journal of Cancer Care,* **11**, 225–31.

Myers, l. (2001) The NHS – a patient's perspective. *Health Expectations,* **4**, 205–8.

Nash, B., Hicks, C. and Dillner, L. (2003) Connecting doctors, patients and the evidence. *British Medical Journal,* **326**, 674.

National Institute for Mental Health in England (2003) *Cases for Change: A Review of the Foundations of Mental Health Policy and Practice, 1997–2002.* National Institute for Mental Health in England, Leeds.

Norman, I. and Peck, E. (1999) Working together in adult community mental health services: an inter-professional dialogue. *Journal of Mental Health,* **8**(3), 217–30.

Onyett, S. (2005) Mental health teams – hitting the targets, missing the point. In: *Beyond the Water Towers* (eds. A. Bell and P. Lindley). Sainsbury Centre for Mental Health, London.

Peck, E. and Norman, I. (1999) Working together in adult community mental health services: exploring inter-professional role relations. *Journal of Mental Health,* **8**(3), 231–42.

Rose, D., Fleischmann, P., Tonkiss, F., Campbell, P. and Wykes, T. (2004) *User and Carer Involvement in Change Management in a Mental Health Context: Review of the Literature.* National Coordinating Centre for NHS Service Delivery and Organisation, London.

Sainsbury Centre for Mental Health (1994) *Relative Values.* Sainsbury Centre for Mental Health, London.

Sainsbury Centre for Mental Health (1997) *Pulling Together: the Future Roles and Training of Mental Health Staff.* Sainsbury Centre for Mental Health, London.

Sainsbury Centre for Mental Health (2000) *Taking Your Partners.* Sainsbury Centre for Mental Health, London.

Silverman, D. (2001) *Interpreting Qualitative Data: Methods for Analysing Talk Text and Interaction.* Sage, London.

Stark, S., Stronach, I. and Warne, T. (2002) Teamwork in mental health: rhetoric and reality. *Journal of Psychiatric and Mental Health Nursing,* **9**, 411–18.

Tailby, S., Richardson, M., Stewart, P., Danford, A. and Upchurch, M. (2004) Partnership at work and worker participation: an NHS case study. *Industrial Relation Journal*, **35**(5), 403–18.

Wildridge, V., Childs, S., Cawthra, L. and Madge, B. (2004) How to create successful partnerships – a review of the literature. *Health Information and Libraries Journal*, **21**, 3–19.

Wensing, M. and Grol, R. (1998) What can patient do to improve health care? *Health Expectations*, **1**, 37–49.

Index